KT-466-543

WITHDRAWN

ALTERNATIVE
MEDICINE:

SHOULD WE SWALLOW IT?

Institute of Ideas
Expanding the Boundaries of Public Debate

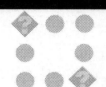

310029

ALTERNATIVE MEDICINE:

SHOULD WE SWALLOW IT?

Institute of Ideas
Expanding the Boundaries of Public Debate

Tiffany Jenkins
Anthony Campbell
Sarah Cant
Bríd Hehir
Michael Fox
Michael Fitzpatrick

Hodder & Stoughton
A MEMBER OF THE HODDER HEADLINE GROUP

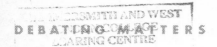
Orders: please contact Bookpoint Ltd, 130 Milton Park, Abingdon, Oxon OX14
4SB. Telephone: (44) 01235 827720. Fax: (44) 01235 400454.
Lines are open from 9.00 - 6.00, Monday to Saturday, with a 24 hour message
answering service. Email address: orders@bookpoint.co.uk

British Library Cataloguing in Publication Data
A catalogue record for this title is available from
the British Library

ISBN 0 340 84838 3

First Published 2002
Impression number   10 9 8 7 6 5 4 3 2 1
Year   2007 2006 2005 2004 2003 2002

Typeset by Transet Limited, Coventry, England.
Printed in Great Britain for Hodder & Stoughton Educational, a division of
Hodder Headline Plc, 338 Euston Road, London NW1 3BH by Cox & Wyman,
Reading, Berks.

CONTENTS

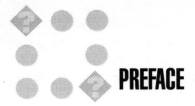

PREFACE

Since the summer of 2000, the Institute of Ideas (IOI) has organized a wide range of live debates, conferences and salons on issues of the day. The success of these events indicates a thirst for intelligent debate that goes beyond the headline or the sound-bite. The IOI was delighted to be approached by Hodder & Stoughton, with a proposal for a set of books modelled on this kind of debate. The *Debating Matters* series is the result and reflects the Institute's commitment to opening up discussions on issues which are often talked about in the public realm, but rarely interrogated outside academia, government committee or specialist milieu. Each book comprises a set of essays, which address one of four themes: law, science, society and the arts and media.

Our aim is to avoid approaching questions in too black and white a way. Instead, in each book, essayists will give voice to the various sides of the debate on contentious contemporary issues, in a readable style. Sometimes approaches will overlap, but from different perspectives and some contributors may not take a 'for or against' stance, but simply present the evidence dispassionately.

Debating Matters dwells on key issues that have emerged as concerns over the last few years, but which represent more than short-lived fads. For example, anxieties about the problem of 'designer babies', discussed in one book in this series, have risen over the past decade. But further scientific developments in reproductive technology, accompanied by a widespread cultural distrust of the implications of these developments, means the debate about 'designer babies' is set to continue. Similarly, preoccupations with the weather may hit the news at times of flooding or extreme weather conditions, but the underlying concern about global warming and the idea that man's intervention into nature is causing the world harm, addressed in another book in the *Debating Matters* series, is an enduring theme in contemporary culture.

At the heart of the series is the recognition that in today's culture, debate is too frequently sidelined. So-called political correctness has ruled out too many issues as inappropriate for debate. The oft noted 'dumbing down' of culture and education has taken its toll on intelligent and challenging public discussion. In the House of Commons, and in politics more generally, exchanges of views are downgraded in favour of consensus and arguments over matters of principle are a rarity. In our universities, current relativist orthodoxy celebrates all views as equal as though there are no arguments to win. Whatever the cause, many in academia bemoan the loss of the vibrant contestation and robust refutation of ideas in seminars, lecture halls and research papers. Trends in the media have led to more 'reality TV', than TV debates about real issues and newspapers favour the personal column rather than the extended polemical essay. All these trends and more have had a chilling effect on debate.

But for society in general, and for individuals within it, the need for a robust intellectual approach to major issues of our day is essential. The *Debating Matters* series is one contribution to encouraging contest about ideas, so vital if we are to understand the world and play a part in shaping its future. You may not agree with all the essays in the *Debating Matters* series and you may not find all your questions answered or all your intellectual curiosity sated, but we hope you will find the essays stimulating, thought provoking and a spur to carrying on the debate long after you have closed the book.

Claire Fox, Director, Institute of Ideas

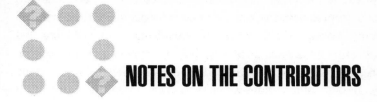

NOTES ON THE CONTRIBUTORS

Anthony Campbell is Emeritus Consultant Physician at The Royal London Homeopathic Hospital, a past director of research at the hospital and past Honorary Editor of the *British Homeopathic Journal*. He was responsible for introducing an acupuncture service at the hospital and has been teaching medical acupuncture to health professionals since 1981. His most recent book is *Acupuncture in Practice: Beyond Points and Meridians* (2001).

Sarah Cant is Senior Lecturer in Applied Social Sciences at Canterbury Christ Church University College. She has written extensively in the areas of medical sociology and health policy and has a particular interest in complementary medicine. Her most recent book is *A New Medical Pluralism, Alternative Medicine, Doctors, Patients and the State* (1999).

Michael Fitzpatrick has been a general practitioner in Hackney, London, for the past 15 years, after training at Oxford University, the Middlesex Hospital and in various hospitals in the London area. He has written on a wide range of medical and political subjects, including AIDS, mad cow disease (and other health scares), drugs and healthcare reform, for both medical publications and the mainstream media. He has also appeared frequently on radio and television and in 1997 produced a critical programme on 'parenting' for the BBC. His book *The Tyranny of Health: Doctors and the Regulation of Lifestyle* was published in 2001.

Michael Fox is the Chief Executive of the Foundation for Integrated Medicine, formed at the personal initiative of His Royal Highness The Prince of Wales, who is now its President. Before joining the Foundation in November 1998, Michael worked in a wide range of roles across the NHS. He has a degree in economics from Trinity College Dublin, and currently chairs London Cyrenians Housing, a charity providing support for people with complex mental health needs.

Bríd Hehir has worked as a nurse for almost 30 years in a number of countries and in a variety of positions – in acute and preventive health care, famine relief, midwifery and health visiting. She graduated with a degree in therapeutic massage from a London University where her exposure to the world of complementary and alternative medicine (CAM) raised concerns in her about the uncritical acceptance by health professionals of the integration of CAM into healthcare in the UK. She is currently employed as a user involvement coordinator with Camden and Islington NHS Trust in London.

Tiffany Jenkins is director of the arts programme at the Institute of Ideas. She is the commissioning editor of the society section of the *Debating Matters* series.

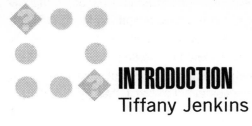

INTRODUCTION
Tiffany Jenkins

Attitudes towards alternative medicine have changed dramatically over the past 20 years. Homeopathy, acupuncture and herbalism, long the preserve of bohemians and eccentrics, are now used by millions as treatments for illness or as part of a healthy lifestyle. Once dismissed by orthodox medicine as harmless fads or dangerous quackery, alternative treatments are now being brought into the mainstream of healthcare. Changing labels reflect the shift in attitudes. In the early 1980s, the term 'alternative' medicine indicated healing traditions that were outside and distinct from conventional medicine. In the 1990s 'alternative' approaches were re-designated as 'complementary' to orthodox medicine. Now the term 'complementary and alternative medicine' (CAM) provides a friendly umbrella under which traditionally rival therapies can shelter. The trend towards 'integrative medicine', which seeks to incorporate some of the principles and practices of CAM into conventional medicine, marks the latest stage in the reconciliation between these historically antagonistic traditions.

At the start of the 1980s health food shops providing information about alternative therapies as well as herbal and other forms of treatment began to appear on the high streets of British cities. Such therapies were at this time outside the mainstream, associated with the radical counterculture or new age mysticism. Yet by the mid-1990s major chain stores had begun to cater for the health-conscious shopper – CAM had become a major retail commodity. Boots the Chemists entered the alternative health market in 1991, offering aromatherapy oils, Bach Flower Remedies and herbal products alongside aspirin and paracetamol, nail varnish and shampoo. In October 2000 Boots extended its range from complementary health products (including vitamins, herbal supplements, aromatherapy and homeopathy) to include, in major branches, consultations on physiotherapy, osteopathy, herbalism, homeopathy, nutrition, aromatherapy and reflexology. In 2001 the supermarket chain Tesco took over the Hale Clinic, an established complementary medicine clinic in London's West End, with prestigious medical consultants and celebrity clients. Tesco now retails Hale Clinic products around the country, guided by the clinic's former proprietor, Rohit Mehta.

Numerous surveys report the rapid expansion in the numbers of people using CAM. A report for the BBC in August 1999, using research commissioned from ICM Research Ltd, showed 21 per cent of the population had used a complementary medicine or therapy in the previous year – double the number found to be using them in a similar survey six years earlier. Britons opting for such therapies spent, on average, almost £15 a month. Citing research commissioned by the Department of Health in 1999, the House of Lords select committee report on CAM found that up to five million patients had consulted a CAM practitioner in the previous year; at least 40 per cent of general practices in the UK provided some CAM services; there were 50,000 CAM practitioners in the UK; and that 10,000 registered health professionals practise some form of CAM (*Complementary and Alternative Medicine: Session 1999– 2000*, 2000). Reflecting this interest, most broadsheet newspapers have a CAM practitioner, such as the Barefoot Doctor in *The Observer*, advising readers on health and lifestyle. Many publishers have created and extended titles to reflect the popularity of alternative therapies. Thorsons, a subsidiary of HarperCollins, spent £500,000 rebranding itself as the leader in this field, a large sum for a niche publisher in UK to spend.

The most dramatic change in attitude towards CAM has taken place within the medical profession. In 1986 the British Medical Association (BMA) published the report *Alternative Therapy*, which indicated a high degree of scepticism about alternative medicine. An attempt to respond to the growing interest in alternatives to conventional medicine, the report's aim was to consider 'the feasibility and possible methods of assessing the value of alternative therapies', and it concluded that for many therapies a formal trial would be impossible. According to the BMA, because alternative medical systems were not based on scientific principles, the scientific method and diagnostic process could not be applied and would be unacceptable to the therapist. While the report stated that there was a need for more research into alternative medicine, this was qualified with the statement that the BMA was committed to orthodox medicine. It was for practitioners of alternative therapies to mount any trial:

> Our long-term duty to our patients is not to support what may be passing fashions, but to ensure for them the benefits of medicine in the future. These include future applications of scientific knowledge; but also, and just as important, orthodox medicine carries the safeguards which arise from entrusting the preservation of health and the care of disease to a registered, recognised and accountable professional, with a long-standing tradition of scientific and personal integrity, including strict standards of confidentiality.

Less than ten years later, in 1993, there was a more conciliatory tone in the BMA's report *Complementary Medicine: New Approaches to Good Practice?* This report recommended a degree of acceptance of some of the more established alternatives to conventional medicine, namely acupuncture, chiropractice, herbal medicine, homeopathy and osteopathy. The report considered a method of regulation for these therapies and discussed 'good practice' guidelines such as registration and training. It recommended that postgraduate students should be taught about these techniques.

The changing attitudes of the medical profession are also evident in comments in leading periodicals such as the *British Medical Journal*. An editorial in 1980 reflected the prevailing hostility of doctors in its characterization of the growing popular interest in alternative medicine as a 'flight from science' (5 January 1980). By 1999, however, the journal was devoting a major series of articles, subsequently published in book form, under the title of the 'ABC' of complementary medicine. In 2001 a special issue, commissioned to coincide with a joint meeting of the British Royal College of Physicians and the US National Center for Complementary and Alternative Medicine, an editorial defined integrated medicine as 'practising medicine in a way that selectively incorporates elements of complementary and alternative medicine into comprehensive treatment plans alongside solidly orthodox methods of diagnosis and treatment' (29 January 2001). Another leading article went so far to suggest that integrating elements of CAM into mainstream medicine could 'restore the soul to medicine'. In another article the director of education for the Royal College of Physicians, Lesley Rees, argued that integrated medicine 'is about restoring core values which have been eroded by social and economic forces. Integrated medicine is good medicine, and its success will be signalled by dropping the adjective. The integrated medicine of today should be the medicine of the new millennium.' In just 20 years, CAM had moved from the margins to take up a place at the centre of the world of orthodox medicine.

Complementary and Alternative Medicine, the 2000 report by a House of Lords select committee and the response from the Government to this report, endorsed the acceptance of CAM. The committee's enquiry was the first comprehensive investigation by a parliamentary body of CAM. The report argued for greater access to CAM, regulation of its practitioners and called for doctors and nurses to recognize the potential of unconventional therapies. The committee advocated that the NHS should make it easier for patients to gain access to CAM therapies and give patients better information about what works and what does not. It drew a distinction between different therapies, by placing them in a first group, for which some evidence of effectiveness was available and which should be regulated; a second group of 'feel good' therapies, which complement conventional medicine and do no harm and for which, significantly, 'proof of treatment-specific effects' was considered less important; or a third group which 'cannot be supported unless and until convincing research evidence of efficacy, based upon the results of well-designed trials, can be produced.' These three groups are as follows:

Group 1: Professionally organized alternative therapies

Acupuncture
Chiropractic
Herbal medicine
Homoeopathy
Osteopathy

Group 2: Complementary therapies

Alexander technique
Aromatherapy
Bach and other flower extracts
Body work therapies, including massage
Counselling stress therapy
Hypnotherapy
Meditation
Reflexology
Shiatsu

Healing
Maharishi ayurvedic medicine
Nutritional medicine
Yoga
Group 3: Alternative disciplines
3a: Long established and traditional systems of healthcare:
Anthroposophical medicine
Ayurvedic medicine
Chinese herbal medicine
Eastern medicine (Tibb)
Naturopathy
Traditional Chinese medicine
3b: Other alternative disciplines:
Crystal therapy
Dowsing
Iridology
Kinesiology
Radionics

The select committee strongly urged medical schools to ensure that all undergraduates are exposed to a level of 'CAM familiarization' and recommended that they consider making optional special study modules in CAM available. The royal colleges were recommended to assist doctors, dentists and veterinary surgeons in familiarizing themselves with CAM therapies through continuing professional development opportunities. It suggested that more research be undertaken and recommended that the NHS and the Medical Research Council provide funding for the development of centres of excellence akin to the National Center for Complementary Medicine in the USA.

Demand for and supply of CAM and its endorsement by influential institutions has been swift and pervasive. But, perhaps surprisingly, this development has generated little debate. Only a few critical voices have been heard either within the medical profession or outside it. Professor Lewis Wolpert, of the Academy of Medical Sciences, is one. In his response to the House of Lords select committee report, he commented that he was 'sorry that any complementary or alternative medicine procedure for which one can see no reasonable scientific basis should be supported.' Before his untimely death from cancer, journalist John Diamond was a vociferous critic. Writing in *The Observer* he stated why he supported orthodox medicine and not CAM:

> The reality is this. For much of the past few hundred years the therapies we now consider alternatives were mainstream. Herbalism has been around for centuries and even the relatively modern homeopathy is almost 300 years old. During all those years people stubbornly continued to die of diseases which are now curable. And then came, modern, orthodox medicine.
>
> And what do you know? People got cured. They stopped dying. They lived longer and enjoyed the life they lived more because they were healthier. Orthodox medicine doesn't have all the answers and can be a force for harm. But much of the time it works. If we're going to spend money on medical research then let it be on improving the stuff we know works rather than on testing remedies which don't.
>
> 3 December 2000

The upsurge in the popularity of CAM and its sudden acceptance by the medical profession needs to be explained. How can we understand the appeal of CAM for patients and doctors – and politicians? What are the consequences of its expansion? There appears to be virtually universal agreement that the integration of CAM and orthodox medicine offers the way forward, but does it? These are some of the questions this book aims to address.

Dr Anthony Campbell, Emeritus Consultant Physician at The Royal London Homeopathic Hospital, provides an overview of the assumptions underlying CAM. He interrogates the claims made by CAM advocates of an affiliation with nature, tradition, and energy. Such claims, for Campbell, may explain the popularity of CAM, because of an emerging disillusionment with the rationality of orthodox medicine. It may be the case, however, that the emperor has no clothes since, argues Campbell, these claims have little foundation.

Sarah Cant, a senior lecturer in applied social sciences at Canterbury Christ Church University College argues that the explanation for the 'renaissance' of alternative therapies is to be found primarily in the consultation room. The demand for CAM has come from the public who have rejected the distant, exclusive and impersonal nature of mainstream medicine. With CAM the patient takes a central and more equal position in the consultation. In this context, contends Cant, they have more control than in their relationship with mainstream medical practitioners. For Cant, the main problem that the increasing regulation of CAM and attempts to 'fit into' mainstream medicine brings is the devaluation of its alternative position which may threaten to reduce its positive qualities.

A 'crisis of confidence' in nursing is the explanation given by Bríd Hehir for the popularity of CAM in the nursing profession. Hehir, who has worked as a nurse for almost 30 years, looks in depth at a specific form of CAM, 'therapeutic touch', developed in the USA and advocated by some nurses in the UK. This therapy, she observes, has been actively embraced by leading figures in the nursing profession and is promoted by them to nurses and the public. Hehir does not welcome the advent of therapeutic touch. It rests, she contends, on a belief system that has no scientific basis and which adopts 'the language of pseudoscience' to attempt to gain credibility. She lambasts it as a deception, which she believes plays on the hopes of ill people offering them relief it cannot possibly hope to achieve.

The following two essays address, from different perspectives, a second issue – the integration of CAM with orthodox medicine in medical practice. Michael Fox, Chief Executive of the Foundation for Integrated Medicine, is a strong advocate of integration. It is here to stay, he argues, because of public demand and the NHS should offer the greatest choice to patients it can. Fox suggests that integrating alternative and orthodox medicines offer the patient 'the best of both worlds'. GP Michael Fitzpatrick argues against integration, contending that the principles and methods of CAM are fundamentally incompatible with those of scientific medicine. Furthermore, he argues that by endorsing CAM orthodox medicine betrays the principles of scientific medicine, principles which have brought enormous benefits to humankind. Fitzpatrick draws attention to the 'loss of nerve' in scientific medicine as a major factor in the rise of CAM. He situates his explanation of the trend towards integration in the context of a society in which medicine has expanded its role far beyond the treatment of disease, defining wider and wider forms of individual and social malaise in medical terms and seeking to regulate personal behaviour in increasingly intrusive and coercive ways. The integration of CAM into orthodox medicine, further endorses the 'medicalization' of troublesome aspects of the contemporary human condition, compounding the problems of individuals and of society.

The essays in this book aim to provide readers with a deeper understanding of some of the issues at stake in the evolution of medicine in the twenty-first century. We hope you find them an insightful contribution to thinking about whether we should swallow complementary and alternative medicine or not.

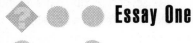

Essay One

COMPLEMENTARY AND ALTERNATIVE MEDICINE: SOME BASIC ASSUMPTIONS
Anthony Campbell

My purpose in this essay is to consider certain basic assumptions or beliefs that underlie much of what is said about complementary and alternative medicine (CAM). I wish to make explicit some of these assumptions in order to try to delineate the differences between two ways of thinking about health and disease. I shall also try to assess how far such concepts stand up to critical evaluation and what they mean for the future of the dialogue between orthodox medicine and CAM.

CAM possesses a certain tone and vocabulary that are recognizably different from those of conventional medicine. Of course, we must be careful about generalizing here. CAM is remarkable for the number and diversity of the therapies that it includes and there are important philosophical differences in attitude within CAM itself; this may not always be appreciated by outside critics. And, as Furnham has argued, it is principally CAM practitioners rather than patients who are influenced by philosophical considerations; patients seeking CAM usually have more practical reasons for doing so (A. Furnham, `Why do people choose and use complementary therapies?' in *Complementary Medicine*, E. Ernst (ed.), 1996).

Within CAM, some practitioners regard unconventional medicine as a set of therapies that can usefully complement orthodox medicine but which make no attempt to replace it, while others are more radical and think that CAM represents a quite different, and better, way of understanding health and disease. It is this second group that I shall principally be concerned with. We could call them advocates of 'alternative' as opposed to 'complementary' medicine. I acknowledge that the difference is relative, not absolute; we are looking at a spectrum of opinion, not a rigid separation into two diametrically opposed positions, but that there is a genuine difference in outlook I have no doubt.

A key feature of the 'alternative' tendency is dissatisfaction with what is perceived to be an excess of rationality in orthodox medicine and this is felt even by some doctors. 'Many of us become interested in acupuncture in part because of a desire to remove ourselves from the excessive rationality of conventional medicine,' writes Dr Michael T. Greenwood ('Acupuncture and intention: needling without needles', *Medical Acupuncture Online Journal*, 11, 1999) and he is certainly not unique among doctors in holding such views. Even mainstream medicine seems to be beginning to accept the view that there is something to be learned from the alternative version. Thus, in a commentary in a recent issue of *Drugs and Therapeutics Bulletin*, we read:

> Traditionally, the establishment has sought to give all it does a scientific base, using science to provide explanations for illness and disease, and for underpinning the development and delivery of management and therapy. However, the expectations of patients are changing. Increasingly, they do not want to be seen as machines in need of repair, but rather as individuals with non-scientific components such as feelings, beliefs and values.

In spite of this rapprochement, however, certain key ideas that characterize much, if not all, of CAM remain difficult to reconcile with orthodox medical thinking. I shall look at four of these, which seem to me to be particularly important. The claims in question are that CAM is (1) natural, (2) traditional, (3) holistic and (4) vitalistic.

THE CONCEPT OF THE NATURAL

One of the commonest claims made on behalf of CAM is that its methods are natural. The word is notoriously difficult to define and indeed it often seems to be used in such a vague way that it amounts to little more than a slogan. This emphasis on the natural is comparatively new. When homeopathy was founded by Samuel Hahnemann in the first half of the nineteenth century little or nothing was said about its being natural. True, the homeopathic remedies advocated by Hahnemann were mainly derived from plants, but so too were those used by his orthodox contemporaries; practically all the medicines in use at the time were herbal. It is only after the development of the modern pharmaceutical industry in the twentieth century that it has made sense to distinguish between natural and synthetic medicines, and even today the difference is not absolute; some important modern drugs are plant derived. At least at its inception, homeopathy differed from 'allopathy', not so much in the materials it used, as in the philosophy on which it was based.

The claim that CAM is natural does not rely wholly on the techniques or on the substances employed. An important part of the idea derives from the supposition that the body (or rather the whole person) has a natural tendency towards health and that it is the function of CAM to facilitate this tendency. In other words, orthodox medicine is thought of as interfering with the system in various ways, all of which are more or less disruptive and unnatural, whereas CAM gently removes blocks that are hindering recovery and allows the natural reparative processes to do their work.

Sensible doctors have always recognized the importance of these natural reparative processes. Penicillin given to a patient with pneumonia may kill the infective organisms but that is not enough, by itself, to bring about recovery; the dead bacteria must be removed and the lungs must be restored to their former healthy state, for example. But the CAM position is more radical than this. CAM holds that our 'natural' state is one of health and that disease is in some sense against nature. We ought not to become ill and in fact we ought not to suffer at all. 'A human being's main and final objective is continuous and unconditional happiness. Any therapeutic system should lead a person towards this objective,' writes G. Vithoulkas, a well-known modern homeopath (*The Science of Homeopathy*, 1980). This hyperbolic tone is not new in homeopathy. In the late-nineteenth century an American homeopath, Charles Hempel, claimed that homeopathy would bring about a complete physical regeneration of mankind that would 'necessarily be attended with great changes in all the external relations of man, education, mode of labouring, living, etc. etc. (preface to S. Hahnemann, *The Chronic Diseases*, trans. C. Hempel, 1845). Statements of this kind sound almost like *The Communist Manifesto*.

Now, quite apart from any doubts we may feel about the ability of CAM to bring about such a total and radical transformation of society as these authors envisage, does the idea that permanent good health is our natural state stand up to serious criticism? I do not think it does. If we take the idea of the natural seriously, it implies that we are the products of Darwinian natural selection. Darwinism is thus central to our understanding of nature, yet its relevance to health and disease has been recognized only recently even within orthodox medicine (A. I. Tauber, 'Darwinian aftershocks: repercussions in the twentieth century', *Journal of the Royal Society of Medicine*, 87: 27–31, 1994) and it is ignored almost totally within CAM. But Darwinism casts considerable doubt on the reassuring belief that our natural state is one of perfect health (R. M. Nesse and G. C. Williams, *Evolution and Healing: The New Science of Darwinian Medicine*, 1995).

The uncomfortable fact is that diseases are entirely natural. In a Darwinian perspective, organisms are continually competing with other organisms for survival. This competition takes many forms but in the present context what matters chiefly is competition with parasites, mainly bacteria and viruses. These alien organisms view us as a free meal and constantly seek to invade us. To resist such alien attacks we have acquired a variety of defence mechanisms during evolution, notably our immune system, and most of the time these mechanisms are amazingly effective. However, they do sometimes fail and sometimes they go wrong and cause damage on their own account: allergies and autoimmune diseases such as rheumatoid arthritis are the result of the immune system becoming overactive or attacking the wrong cells. Cancer has been described by Charlton as a form of 'endogenous parasitism' ('Senescence, cancer, and endogenous parasites: a salutogenic hypothesis', *Journal of the Royal College of Physicians*, 30: 10–12, 1996). Both immunology and genetics, two branches of science which seem certain to revolutionize our understanding of disease, are Darwinian through and through,

The belief that our natural state is to be healthy all the time is at best a half-truth and one that slides rather easily into sentimentality. The mistake is to confuse general statistical trends with the fate of individuals. Natural selection works statistically; it offers no guarantee that a given individual will not come to grief. Disease, degeneration and unlucky draws in the genetic lottery are part of life and it is profoundly misleading to suggest that anything we may do can make us immune to them. One of the worst features of CAM, in my view, is that it may lead people to adopt an overoptimistic expectation of their prospects for health that is liable to end in disappointment and a feeling of betrayal.

◆ ● ●
● ● ● **COMPLEMENTARY AND ALTERNATIVE MEDICINE**
● ● ◆ **AS TRADITION**

As Rosalind Coward has pointed out (*The Whole Truth*, 1989), hardly any form of CAM makes a point of claiming to be entirely new. On the contrary, those disciplines that are indubitably antique, such as herbalism, traditional Chinese medicine and Ayurvedic medicine, emphasize the fact as lending them enhanced legitimacy and even systems of more recent origin, such as homeopathy, often claim to have antecedents in the writings of Hippocrates and other early sages. If a system is supposed to be traditional, however, it must also be relatively static and unchanging. Far from seeing this as a weakness, supporters of such systems generally make a virtue of the fixed nature of their ideas, which are described as immutable principles. Thus Harris Coulter writes that 'the homeopathy doctrine [sic] is stable and has never suffered the upheavals of rationalist medicine' (*Homeopathic Science and Modern Medicine*, 1980).

But it is precisely these 'upheavals' that constitute the advancement of scientific knowledge, while 'doctrines' are appropriate for religions but not for science. This distinction is clearly understood by Kaptchuk in relation to acupuncture. Traditional Chinese medicine, he says, is pre-scientific, because it is unchanging:

> The ancient books are the language of Chinese medicine, and while the vocabulary can be expanded and enriched, the grammar and syntax are fixed. Complete and self-contained, traditional Chinese medicine is incapable of assimilating anything that challenges its fundamental assumptions.
> *Chinese Medicine: The Web That Has No Weaver*, 1983

Similar remarks could be applied to most if not all types of CAM. In this important respect they differ sharply from orthodox medicine, which since the mid-nineteenth century has been founded on science and has changed progressively as science has changed. The most basic feature of science is that it proceeds by continually questioning its own assumptions. CAM systems, in contrast, can never question their basic assumptions, for then they would be sawing off the branch on which they are sitting.

HOLISM

The claim that CAM is holistic is pretty well universal among its practitioners (D. Peters, 'Is complementary medicine holistic?' in *Examining Complementary Medicine*, A. Vickers (ed.), 1998). 'Holistic', like 'natural', is a rather vague term which seems to mean different things to different people, but the basis is usually taken to be the idea that CAM 'treats the patient as a whole person'. The length of the consultation is often taken as an index of this. CAM practitioners typically spend a long time with their patients, often 45 minutes or an hour, and sometimes longer. This affords the opportunity to discuss a wide range of issues and patients undoubtedly appreciate this. Orthodox doctors generally say that they would like to spend more time with their patients too, but pressure of time and lack of resources within the National Health Service often make it difficult or impossible. An important reason why CAM practitioners can provide more time for their patients is that most of them work in private practice. Homeopathic doctors who work within the National Health Service at NHS hospitals often complain that they are unable to give as much time to their patients as they would like. Even allowing for this difference, however, it is certainly true to say that most CAM practitioners give their patients more time than do most orthodox doctors.

8

But how is this extra time used? In many cases, CAM practitioners are looking at what they regard as important causes of disease. They generally pay more attention to lifestyle, diet, and emotional questions than do orthodox doctors and such matters form an important aspect of the 'holistic' approach to disease. This emphasis accords with what many patients are now seeking. Patients who come for alternative medicine frequently say: 'I don't want just to take a drug to suppress my symptoms, I want to find the cause', and we constantly hear claims by CAM practitioners that conventional medicine merely deals with the superficial manifestations of disease instead of eradicating it at the root, as CAM is supposed to do. On the face of it this is rather strange, for if you asked most orthodox doctors what they think of alternative medicine their main criticism would be that it is merely a placebo that may help on a symptomatic level but does not tackle the causes of disease. We are therefore confronted with the curious paradox that both sets of practitioners believe themselves to be treating the causes of disease while their opponents are merely offering palliatives. The explanation is that the two groups have different ideas about what counts as a cause.

Since the middle of the nineteenth century, if not longer, the trend towards thinking of the body as a very complicated machine, but a machine nonetheless, has been becoming ever stronger in medicine. Even psychiatry, for long the one exception to this, is today almost wholly mechanistic; modern psychiatry is pretty much a branch of neurology and psychiatric disorders are thought of as brain diseases (editorial, *The Lancet*, 244:681–82, 1994). And this trend has received a huge impetus from recent discoveries in genetics and molecular biology, which have shown that there is a mechanistic explanation for many of the most basic processes of life. For orthodox medicine, the key to understanding disease is pathology. That is, orthodox doctors do not feel confident that they have really understood a disease until they can give a detailed account of it at the cellular and, ideally, the molecular level.

CAM practitioners, in contrast, are comparatively uninterested in pathology, which they consider to be of secondary importance. These mechanisms may exist, they concede, but we need not get caught up in them. Much of CAM is therefore concerned with identifying factors in patients' lives that predispose them to becoming ill. The 'real' causes of disease are, for example, obscure and subtle deficiencies in diet, food allergies, disturbances in the 'primary rhythm' of cerebrospinal circulation, 'geopathic stress', 'candida', miasms and numerous other factors that do not figure in mainstream science. The various CAM systems have different explanatory schemes but all share similar functions: to provide a label for the patient's symptoms which is psychologically satisfying and to suggest a course of treatment – naturally, one that is appropriate for the practitioner in question to supply. An important aspect of such explanations is that they do not depend on complex ideas like those of modern molecular biology; even if they are superficially technological, as in the case of supposed mineral or vitamin deficiencies, the principles are easy to grasp even for patients with minimal scientific knowledge.

In keeping with such ideas is the oft repeated claim that CAM 'treats the person, not the disease'. Much is made of this in homeopathy, where the prescription in cases of chronic disease is generally arrived at on the basis of 'constitution'. Patients are asked about their fears, their food likes and dislikes, their climatic preferences and other matters, none of which may have any direct connection with the symptoms of which they are complaining. Homeopaths like to emphasize the fact that two patients with the same pathological diagnosis may receive different homeopathic prescriptions.

The 'holistic' value of such methods is, however, debatable. The conceptual basis of the diagnoses that are arrived at is often quite narrow. In the case of homeopathy, for example, the questions asked are usually fairly stereotypical and the remedy prescribed is often selected from a fairly small range of possibilities; it usually turns out to be one of the 'polychrests', of which there are perhaps about 20 or even fewer. There is nothing surprising about this; the polychrests are so called because they are associated with a particularly large number of symptoms, so it is to be expected that they will in fact be the remedies that are commonly pointed to by the consultation.

The majority of CAM practitioners use only a small selection from the available range of treatments. For example, a homeopath may well know little or nothing about herbal medicines apart from the relatively few that also happen to be homeopathic remedies, while an acupuncturist may have no experience of osteopathy or an osteopath of acupuncture, even though both acupuncture and osteopathy are manual treatments and probably work in quite similar ways. It may be unreasonable to expect most practitioners to have trained in more than one or perhaps two different forms of treatment, but it is not unreasonable to expect that they should at least have an idea of the limitations of what they themselves offer and some knowledge of the alternatives that exist; however, this is often not the case. Real holistic treatment, I suggest, would consist in knowing a good deal about the scope and limitations of most of the treatments available, including orthodox treatment, together with a willingness to refer the patient to whichever practitioner seemed most likely to help. This ideal is not always achieved in practice.

It could indeed be said with some plausibility that the setting of CAM tends if anything to militate against holism in the sense just described. Because most CAM practice is in the private sector the practitioners often work alone and even if they share premises with others they seldom meet regularly to discuss difficult cases and compare notes. In hospitals, in contrast, meetings of this kind involving doctors, physiotherapists, nurses and others are routine, generally held weekly and are prescribed as part of audit. Such meetings provide the opportunity to learn about other health professionals' approaches and expertize and to explore the different possibilities for treatment that may be available (A. Vickers, 'Criticism, scepticism and complementary medicine', in *Examining Complementary Medicine*, A. Vickers (ed.), 1998).

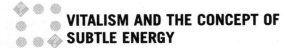

VITALISM AND THE CONCEPT OF SUBTLE ENERGY

It is difficult to read much about CAM without coming across references to 'energy'. This is really a modern way of naming something that used to be called the life force and was taken seriously by at least some scientists as recently as the early twentieth century. Its origins are probably prehistoric. In earlier times it was generally held that there is some kind of subtle substance or force that is responsible for life. This principle was often identified with the breath, doubtless because we only stop breathing when we are dead. This might be conceived of in a fairly literal way, so that the soul was thought of as escaping from the dying body in the last breath. In Greek, *pneuma* refers both to breath and to spirit and the same idea is found in the Sanskrit word *prana*. The corresponding Chinese concept is *qi*, often rendered as 'energy' in western texts. In oriental schemes such as the so-called meridians of acupuncture or the chakras of ancient Indian subtle anatomy, this energy is supposed to flow in particular channels or pathways.

Belief in the vital force persisted in European medicine at least until the eighteenth century, when it was favoured at the University of Montpellier in the south of France. Samuel Hahnemann, although initially scornful of the idea, later introduced it to homeopathy where it became enshrined as a central part of its founder's dogma. The process of 'dynamization', consisting in the pattern of alternate dilution and violent shaking (succussion) which Hahnemann invented to make the medicines, was explained by him in terms of the vital force; indeed, we could think of homeopathic medicines as the vital force captured in a bottle.

The actual term 'vital force' is probably used less frequently in CAM today but 'energy' is the modern equivalent. Many forms of CAM, including radionics, dowsing and crystal therapy all base themselves on ideas of energy and even the manipulative therapies make use of the idea at times. The oriental systems, especially acupuncture, have it as a central concept; acupuncture is often said to depend on 'energy balancing' that adjusts the flow of *qi* in the meridians. As a concept, 'energy' is meaningful to many people. Colloquially, we describe a person as having much or little energy and we say that we are 'low in energy' when we feel disinclined to work. The idea thus works well at a psychological or emotional level; it functions adequately as a metaphor. But it is when we take the metaphor literally and claim that this energy is real and objective in the same way that electromagnetic energy is real that the problems arise.

If we ask detailed questions about the nature and function of this subtle energy we find, as Wood has said, 'total confusion' (C. Wood, 'Subtle energy and the vital force in complementary medicine', in *Examining Complementary Medicine*, A. Vickers, (ed.), 1998). There is no agreement about what it is or how it functions. Indeed, there is seldom any serious attempt to describe the operations of energy in any detail. There have been attempts to update the concept by reference to contemporary physics, but these rarely amount to more than vague analogies. There are also claims that modern research methods are capable of actually demonstrating the existence of subtle energy – Kirlian photography is a popular tool for doing this – but the experimental evidence is generally unconvincing except to people who already believe in the concept for other reasons. All this is a good example of what Richard Feynman called cargo cult science – theories and experiments that have the outward form of science but lack what is really essential to make it work.

I agree with Wood that the concepts of 'energy' and 'energy medicine', though popular with many CAM practitioners, have no real intellectual content. 'Energy' in this context is a metaphor, no more, albeit one that works for many practitioners and their patients. It thus has a use within its own context, but it also makes those forms of CAM that employ it more remote than they would otherwise be from mainstream science. However, not all CAM practitioners find this separation important; some even welcome it. For the more extreme among them, orthodox medicine is not merely narrow-minded and misguided, it is actually dangerous, and the sooner it is completely rebuilt on a different model, the better.

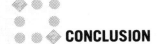

CONCLUSION

I have touched on a number of features of CAM that distinguish it conceptually from orthodox medicine. Attachment to such ideas is really an aspect of a deeper problem with CAM, which is the question of how it is supposed to work. Although research has provided a limited amount of evidence for the efficacy of some forms of CAM, including acupuncture, homeopathy, osteopathy and chiropractic, it has been difficult to provide plausible mechanisms for them. Medical acupuncturists have responded by largely abandoning the traditional form and constructing new models based on modern anatomy and physiology; there have been rather similar trends within osteopathy and chiropractic. Homeopathy is at present almost wholly without a plausible explanatory basis, a failing that has delayed its acceptance by orthodox medicine. If and when these forms of CAM become incorporated into orthodox practice they will need to be equipped with a scientific rationale of some kind, but this will inevitably eliminate many of the features that give CAM its distinctive character. There is a paradox here that may not be easy to resolve.

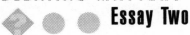

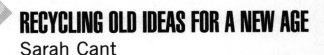

RECYCLING OLD IDEAS FOR A NEW AGE
Sarah Cant

A short history of medicine

'I have an earache ...'

2000 BC	Here, eat this root.
1000 AD	That root is heathen. Here, say this prayer.
1850 AD	That prayer is superstition. Here, drink this potion.
1940 AD	That potion is snake oil. Here, swallow this pill.
1985 AD	That pill is ineffective. Here take this antibiotic.
2000 AD	That antibiotic is artificial. Here, eat this root.

(Anonymous)

The traditional history of medicine tells a story of great men who, with the help of science, overthrew charlatanry and quackery. The humoral theory, which described the body as consisting of four bodily fluids each responding to four elements in the universe, experienced a remarkably long period of success until science penetrated deeper into the body and its folly was revealed. It is an Hegelian account of rupture, one paradigm replaced by another in the triumphal story of progress. Yet, if science, discovery and progress are the keys to understanding the advance of medical knowledge, why has there been the renaissance of alternative and traditional medicines and a return to the past?

16

THE LIMITS OF BIOMEDICINE

The history of medicine provides us with a barometer by which to gauge social and cultural change. The power of religion and its subsequent decline has been central to the development of many healthcare practices. The anatomist, doctor and artist Versalius (1514–64) may never have robbed graves and dissected bodies had the process of secularization not begun. And yet, as we shall see, the importance of the spirit in understanding health and disease has not entirely faded. Of course, it was the Enlightenment period that became so important for the development of what we now term 'modern' medicine. Its philosophical underpinnings allowed the Cartesian split of the mind and spirit from the body and the body itself became a site for experimentation. Science heralded progress and an optimism that the ills of society might be eradicated. This could have been an end to the story. Certainly the success of biomedicine in the twentieth century, particularly the control of acute disease, seemed to guarantee permanence and stability and doctors, of all the professionals, attracted absolute public esteem. They did the most good, working altruistically and objectively to cure illness and prevent disease. Yet, plainly, this image is no longer a popular one. We know that doctors make mistakes, are often uncertain about diagnosis and treatment and have not been able to provide the magic bullet for many chronic and disabling diseases. The promise of scientific knowledge has not always delivered and, in some cases, it has brought as many problems as solutions.

The power of biomedicine then cannot lie entirely in the success of the knowledge base. Medical sociologists have partly explained the rise of biomedicine in terms of the ability of doctors to professionalize.

They organized themselves internally, establishing social closure through the creation of extensive training programmes and credentials. The medical profession became very exclusive, preventing, for many years, women from even entering the training programmes. With strong social status and the promise of scientific knowledge the medical profession adeptly managed to secure the support of the state, and in turn, a monopolistic position. These strategies have left an important legacy.

According to the humoral theory of medicine, the mind, spirit and body were important for an understanding of ill health and therefore the patients' own interpretations and understandings of their symptoms were critical. Moreover, before medicine had secured its monopoly of the healthcare market, it had had to compete with many other healing traditions and the patients, or more accurately consumers, chose and paid for the services they desired. Thus, in the nineteenth century the bedside manner of the doctor was critical, the relationship with the doctor being as important as the actual medicines that were being dispensed. Biomedical practitioners have worked to change this relationship with their patients. In particular, the social distance between doctors and patients has increased, bestowing the doctor a more powerful position, one that stands above lay scrutiny and judgement. The growing efficacy of biomedicine and the development of the hospital saw the patient become less important. Scientific tests rather than face-to-face communication gave answers to medical conundrums and the patients' understanding and emotions were designated much lower priority, so much so that one might argue that the patient became docile in the healing process.

Until relatively recently Britain supported a plural medical market. In the early part of the twentieth century people could still choose from a vast array of healing systems and practitioners. Yet the burgeoning

18

success of biomedicine also bestowed the power to resolve the problem of competitors in the healthcare market. Nurses and midwives were subordinated, dentists and opticians limited in their practice and other knowledge systems were either absorbed (some homeopathic remedies, for example) or discredited and excluded. The *British Medical Journal* is filled with assaults on what we only now label *alternative* medicine. Biomedical practitioners who chose to provide homeopathy, for instance, were publicly chastised. By the time the National Health Service was established, providing healthcare free at the point of delivery, only homeopathy survived and then only in a tokenistic way.

Considering the dominance of the biomedical profession, their support from the state and pharmaceutical companies, it is surprising that alternative medicines have experienced a revival. Yet, despite cost disincentives (most alternative medicine is purchased in the private sector), consumers are increasingly turning to other practitioners and knowledge bases. Any quick scan of the health section of the local bookshop, the range of remedies available in the chemist, the number of articles in magazines and newspapers, is testimony to a significant turn in the healthcare practices of the lay populace. Mothers are applying arnica to their children's bruises; we are detoxing our bodies; going to yoga classes; visiting the chiropractor or osteopath for our lower back pain; using acupuncture to aid weight loss and smoking cessation; and using a variety of practitioners to alleviate the symptoms of HIV or provide a miracle cure for cancer. Although the survey data are problematic (different populations have been surveyed and different therapies considered) we know that about a third of the population have used some form of alternative medical care (this includes self-medication) and that a quarter of the population have visited a practitioner. Although women are more likely to visit a practitioner than men and the middle classes more than the working classes (the money issue must be a factor here) there are no other significant demographic differences between users and non-users. There is some evidence that users are more health conscious than non-users, are more likely to have a chronic illness and are less likely to smoke or drink. However, it is not true that users are more hypochondriacal than the average population, neither are they vegans who wear plastic shoes. Using alternative medicine is not a marginal exercise; it is something we all might contemplate.

EXPLAINING THE RENAISSANCE OF ALTERNATIVE MEDICINE

It is more accurate to talk of alternative medicines than alternative medicine, as non-biomedical modes of healing cannot be understood as a single category. Therapies differ in the extent to which they portray themselves as having complete systems of treatment, whether they are regulated, whether they have a strong evidence base and so on. There are at least 160 different therapies on offer. These therapies have either been imported by westerners in various versions from Asia (for example acupuncture), have entered western countries with immigrant groups (such as Unani Tibb, Ayurveda, Chinese herbal medicine, various forms of spiritual healing), have found a new popularity after a period of eclipse (homeopathy, herbalism) or have been introduced from America (osteopathy, chiropractic, reflexology). Thus, for the most part, these modes of healing are not new, having their origins in various moments in the history of healing. Moreover, many of these healing practices do not stand outside biomedicine; for example, homeopathy and acupuncture are now widely practised by doctors. The absorption of competitive ideas is not new to biomedicine but why did these forms of knowledge become so popular, when many are untested and are based on ideas that make no sense to modern science? For example, homeopathy works on the principles of 'like cures like' and that the remedies should be so diluted that they can no longer be traced, thus contradicting all laws of chemistry. Indeed, some practitioners will admit that they do not know why their therapy works. The return to alternative medicines is not just about the plausibility or scientificity of its knowledge bases.

To understand the popularity of alternative medicine we must first enter the consultation room. In the majority of encounters within alternative medicine it is likely that the patient will take a central position, having the opportunity to provide information about their health status. The holistic emphasis of much alternative medicine requires that patients give an extensive personal history and engage with the emotional and spiritual dimensions of illness episodes (of course, this is not true of all consultations with an osteopath for instance and even in homeopathy not all patients are prepared to divulge all the information a practitioner may ask for). Such an approach to healthcare demands a more individualistic response to patients and, in turn, patients are elevated to expert status, critical players in the understanding of their health. Overall, patients seem to enjoy having more control and participation and can come to see a practitioner as much as a confidante and friend as a healer. It is also the case that many consultations within alternative medicine work to help the patient make sense of their own illness by linking it to a range of wider cultural, personal and social frameworks. For example, an alternative medical practitioner will require an extensive family history and will spend a long time questioning patients about their lifestyle and environment. This is in stark contrast to many of the reductionist accounts used by orthodox medicine.

To achieve a mutual and sharing relationship between the patient and practitioner and so engender good bedside manner, of course, requires time. Within the National Health Service, doctors are overworked and cannot offer the hour-long consultations that alternative practitioners can provide. Thus, some of the attractions of alternative medicine are rooted in the dynamics and meaning of the consultation and others in its structure, aspects that orthodox medicine may do well to reflect upon.

This is not to say that the effectiveness of alternative medicine does not play a part in its attractiveness to patients. Surveys of users have found widespread satisfaction with alternative medicine and the majority claim to experience an improvement to their condition. The majority of patients use alternative medicine for chronic and intractable conditions, notably those conditions where the orthodox medical profession has had the least success. While some of the biomedical establishment may be at pains to explain any improvement in terms of the placebo effect or may assert that the medical conditions seen by alternative practitioners are self-limiting, the same argument can, of course, be levelled at orthodox medicine itself. I am not in a position to judge the efficacy or otherwise of alternative medicine. It is true that there has been very little research but neither has there been any money forthcoming to conduct the research and alternative practitioners are not in a position to fund huge randomized control trials (many cannot sustain an income for themselves). This is aside from the fact that some alternative practitioners do not see scientific research methods as the best way to evaluate their practice. For instance, there have been problems when the collaboration between general practitioners and alternative practitioners has been evaluated. The alternative practitioners complain that they are referred the so-called 'heart-sink' patients, those for whom orthodox medicine cannot offer any more help. In turn, the alternative practitioners are judged to have failed when the client does not show significant improvement. There is nothing wrong with judging and evaluating alternative medicine so long as it is done equitably and appropriately.

Our society is one that has become obsessed with health. We are bombarded with information about diets and exercise and about self-improvement. In this context of 'healthism', it is not surprising that alternative medicines have become more popular. In fact, all the evidence shows that it is a minority of people who opt out of biomedicine in favour of alternative medicines. Instead there has been a multiplication of health practices, patients using orthodox medicine alongside alternative medicines. In search of the perfect body and perfect health, we are in the gym, at the doctors, eating healthy food and visiting a variety of other practitioners. Health-related behaviour has become a central activity in the twenty-first century and a huge consumer market (the Royal Pharmaceutical Society estimated that £93 million was spent on alternative medicines in 1998). Alternative medicine, as distinct from biomedicine (although biomedicine has this potential), is more concerned with the promotion of good health, rather than the alleviation of ill health. Stable users (those that go to see alternative practitioners on a regular basis) are very likely to incorporate the promotion of 'good health' as part of their explanations for seeking advice. There is some evidence that users of alternative medicine are more likely to believe that their health can be improved and are generally more knowledgeable about their bodies, although this may be a product of the educative potential of many alternative therapies. Some of the users of alternative medicine seek care for conditions that would not be defined as illness in the biomedical sense. For example, reflexology can be used to aid relaxation and enhance feelings of well-being.

Consequently, the increased use of alternative medicines forces us to redefine our understanding of what actually constitutes healthcare practices. Where healthcare has been traditionally equated with medical techniques of the body, it may now need to broaden to include all those recreational and aesthetic techniques that the consumer links to 'feeling healthy'. These are important political definitions as it is unlikely that the NHS could stretch to provide for such consultations, even if they do contribute to qualitative measures of 'good' health.

There are arguments to suggest that both alternative and orthodox practitioners work to medicalize and control our every move. Aspects of our lives that used to stand outside medical intervention are now understood in terms of health and illness. Our children are not badly behaved, they suffer from attention deficit syndrome; to cope with the menopause we must take a range of vitamin supplements before onset and have HRT afterwards. But we, the consumers, also want these 'medical ' definitions – our babies cry only because of their traumatic delivery and need to be seen by a cranial osteopath. We have increasingly high expectations of ourselves and the way we should lead our lives and we require an expert to help us seek out explanations for any of our imperfections. This is not to say there is no foundation to any of these complaints, but they are not new. Our tolerance has changed, the result of differing needs, values and expectations.

It is also the case that the general public has become disillusioned with biomedical science. Medical science had promised progress and predictability but the increased knowledge of risks associated with medical intervention have served to temper the optimism for biomedicine and fuelled a need to search for safer and less artificial alternatives. There has been in some sense a return to 'nature' (although there is plenty of evidence to show that some alternative medicines are far from safe or natural). Many studies show that users of alternative medicine are concerned about the side-effects of drugs and are anxious about taking medication that seems to them to be made from artificial substances and chemicals. The apparent harmlessness of alternative medicine and its association with natural and organic products stands as an important attraction. There is a sense in which the product rather than the knowledge base is important here.

Part of the questioning of orthodox science has come from the publicity about its mistakes but also because the lay public, aided by the internet and media, has become more knowledgeable and critical. While *Casualty* and *ER* glamorize the medical profession, there are as many documentaries that question the objectivity and safety of modern medicine. Consumers are not prepared to accept medical advice at face value, but instead will explore the possibilities of their condition and the variety of alternatives possible. To be a medical expert, to have credentials and strong internal organization, is no longer enough to engender trust. Perhaps we are just more vocal about our mistrust of the medical profession – many of us never did take our prescriptions – so our access to biomedical and alternative knowledges has made our scepticism more explicit and legitimate.

The increased knowledgeability and reflexivity of the patient has produced a situation where the expertise of the biomedical practitioner is no longer guaranteed. But this critical stance also extends itself to alternative medicine. Consumers (as well as the medical profession and government) want to know that practitioners are trained, safe and accountable as well as caring and understanding. When alternative medicine first experienced its revival in the late 1970s the therapists had, on the whole, not attended training courses and did not belong to professional organizations. Taking homeopathy as an example, this therapy had continued to be practised by medical doctors on a small scale throughout the twentieth century. Medical homeopathy took on a particular complexion, practised alongside allopathic medicine. However, two non-medically qualified practitioners, Da Monte and Maughan, who were also druids, took an interest in the homeopathic principles. The homeopathic healing practices were consequently incorporated into their druidic philosophy and these charismatic men passed on their teachings to interested followers. There was no structure to the teaching or a curriculum, rather these men would talk about homeopathy alongside other bodies of knowledge, far removed from the teachings of medical homeopathy. There was great emphasis placed upon the spirituality of homeopathy, the vital force and upon constitutional/individualized prescribing. In contrast, the medically qualified homeopaths were more likely to use 'pathological' prescribing, where the choice of remedy was chosen on the basis of the disease category from which the patient suffered, rather than the patient's individual constitution.

Non-medically qualified homeopathy thus emerged as a highly individualistic movement and placed emphasis on an interactive and non-hierarchical relationship with the patient. It was a radical and charismatic revival, indeed some therapists held the view that their form of treatment would eventually supersede biomedicine. However, pressures from the medical profession (a player I return to later), the Government and consumers meant that this form of practice could not be sustained. The non-medically qualified homeopaths were also concerned that an increasing number of people were 'dabbling' with the homeopathy they gleaned from books. Thus there was a recognition that the practitioners must organize internally and transmit their knowledge in a codified and exclusive way. In other words they needed to portray themselves as experts, with a monopoly over their knowledge – they needed to professionalize.

The 1980s thus saw the formulation of syllabi, credentials and registers of competent practitioners within many therapy groups. There are now hundreds of training colleges in Britain and it is estimated that there are over 50,000 therapists. It is now possible to read for degrees in osteopathy, chiropractic, homeopathy and herbalism. Training colleges have core curricula, standardized training and clear entry requirements (although the standards vary tremendously by therapy group). The process of social closure of the alternative medical professions is thus well under way. Professional bodies judge which practitioners are competent and use disciplinary procedures if the agreed code of ethics is transgressed. While alternative medicine might be about individualized treatment and non-hierarchical relations with patients, it has also become about boundaries of expertise. The way in which therapists train and practise has thus changed immeasurably, becoming to look more and more like biomedicine and it will be interesting to see whether this may, in the longer term, fail to sustain interest from the consumers.

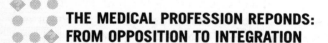

THE MEDICAL PROFESSION REPONDS: FROM OPPOSITION TO INTEGRATION

The medical profession, as we might expect, was wary about the renaissance of alternative medicines and indeed the degree of interest taken in alternative knowledges by some of its own practitioners. The first response was to try to discredit these popular knowledges on the basis of their lack of scientificity and safety. The British Medical Association report of 1986 was a vitriolic attack. The first 34 of its 161 pages consisted of an account of the progressive development of modern biomedicine as a scientific discipline. Some of the main forms of alternative medicine were then discussed, with an assessment of any scientific evidence for their efficacy. The conclusion was that doctors could not feel confident about alternative medicine and that patients should be protected from treatments that had not been scientifically validated and were potentially harmful.

This discreditation exercise was, in fact, a failure, meeting with public disdain and criticism from many doctors within the establishment. Thus, in 1990 another working party was set up with a much less damaging agenda. The report wanted to provide suitable medical guidance for the consumer and concentrated not on the scientific basis of alternative medicines but their competence to practise. It talked of doctors providing alternative medicine and working alongside other practitioners. It is, of course, possible to interpret this as a strategy of absorption. Moreover, while the increasing interest by medical practitioners in alternative medicine should be welcomed, there is some danger that the actual provision of the therapies may change. Will acupuncture simply become more widely available as more general practitioners are trained to provide it (accessing those who currently are unable to pay)? Or will this form of acupuncture be very different? There is some evidence to suggest that we might see a medicalized form of acupuncture (sometimes called 'needling') which uses formula needle points for a number of clearly defined and restricted conditions. If the vital extract of a valuable herb can be turned into tablet form, will it still be effective and will the transaction between the practitioner and patient be as satisfactory? And, if doctors are to provide alternative medicines, what demands need to placed on their levels of training and regulation?

It is interesting that although the medical profession failed to discredit alternative medicines, an impact of their concern has been that many alternative medical organizations have made the public claims for their therapy less radical. Non-medically qualified homeopaths, for instance, have dropped their anti-vaccination stance, the chiropractors only make claims to alleviate back pain rather than cure organic disease and most therapists see their role as complementary rather than alternative to biomedicine. This rapprochement has paved the way for collaboration and integration. There have been increasing instances of alternative medicines being brought into the NHS (although this is very cash bound and dependent on the attitudes of the primary care group). It is interesting, however, that while these projects offer financial security to practitioners they also start to change the way in which alternative medicine is practised. In particular, it is possible that alternative practitioners may only be referred certain types of patients and complaints, so losing their holistic approach and constrained to fit into the much shorter NHS consultation slots. There is a sense in which alternative medicines will become more and more like biomedicine and in doing so their appeal may be curtailed.

There is another important way in which alternative medicine has been forced to change. In Britain both the National Government and the European Union have taken an interest in the growth of alternative medicine. For the European Union, the new found popularity of alternative medicine is hugely problematic, not least because the member states all have very different policies. The operation of Napoleonic law in some European countries restricts much alternative medical practice to doctors, whereas in Britain, common law allows all forms of medicine, as long as the therapist does not call herself a doctor. From the 1990s the British Government took a more interventionist stance towards complementary medicine, requiring that therapy groups work towards the regulation of their professions. This can take place via self- or statutory regulation. Both osteopathy and chiropractic have state regulation (it is likely that herbalism, acupuncture and homeopathy will soon follow suit) and this has afforded them a monopoly, an exclusive right to provide their therapy. Thus the state has stepped in to assure patients about the expertise of their practitioners (state regulation was dependent on showing high degrees of training and professional organization). In doing so, certain groups have been bestowed a form of legitimacy and this has, in turn, created a hierarchy within alternative medicine. The more 'legitimate' therapies are those that are most likely to collaborate with general practice. The other therapy groups are being encouraged to engage in voluntary self-regulation, to extend their training and find proof of their effectiveness. While these are important milestones in the establishment of trust they are difficult to achieve. If spiritual healing is a gift, how can it be taught? How can smaller groups establish research training programmes? It is likely that some therapies will retreat to the fringe of the healthcare market.

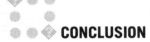

CONCLUSION

The return to alternative medicine has been as much about a yearning for a different type of relationship with a practitioner as a search for cure. Undoubtedly, alternative medicines use different knowledges and treatments and have successes but we learn that the process of care is as important as the outcome. Patients need to feel part of the consultation, to be an equal participant in the healing process. A reflective orthodox profession might look to its own form of practice and contemplate the bedside manner of the past and the involvement of the patient in decisions. In times of uncertainty over medical diagnosis and treatment, absolving some of the responsibility to the patient may be no bad thing. But, it is more than this. Chronically ill patients need attention given to their emotional and social needs as well as their bodily ones – holistic medicine is nothing more than good medical practice. The philosophies of alternative medicine resonate with our changing cultural demands. But these are conflictual demands. We desire a caring, participative and meaningful relationship with our therapists but also want them to prove their expertise and trustworthiness. History has taught us that in establishing expertise the doctors also established distance. This is especially likely if alternative medicine is to be integrated further into the NHS. While the increased accessibility of alternative medicines should be welcomed, shorter consultations, the referral of patients from the general practitioner and thus increased pathological rather than individualized prescribing may change the practice of alternative medicines immeasurably. The challenge for alternative medicine will be to retain its appeal, extend its accessibility and prove its worthiness to practise.

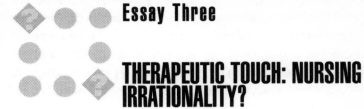

Essay Three

THERAPEUTIC TOUCH: NURSING IRRATIONALITY?
Bríd Hehir

Nursing interest in complementary and alternative medicine (CAM) in Britain has increased in recent years and CAM has now become an acceptable, even expected, part of nurses' repertoire of skills. This development is paralleled by public demand for CAM. What was once rare has become passé and everyday, for example, massage, reflexology, homeopathy and osteopathy. Therapeutic touch (TT), which this essay will look at in some depth, is a relatively new girl on the block and is being promoted to British healthcare workers, nurses in particular, as a positive intervention that will benefit practitioners and recipients. TT is a form of 'energy healing' that can apparently trigger extraordinary clinical, social and even miraculous effects. At one level it is reported to promote relaxation, to decrease anxiety levels, to reduce the perception of pain and to facilitate healing. Work by its founder, Delores Krieger suggested that premature babies who had been extubated and left for dead were resuscitated through TT (D. P. O'Mathúna, *Scientific Review of Alternative Medicine*, 1998). It has also been reported to be a social force that has brought together Israelis and Egyptians along the Gaza Strip. It has been used in emergency situations such as the terrorist bombing in Oklahoma City (J. A. Straneva, 'Therapeutic touch coming of age', *Holistic Nursing Practice*, 14 (3): 2000). More recently, the Nurse Healers Association advised its membership, after the 2001 World Trade Center explosions, to heal people at a distance, to visualize themselves at a person's side performing TT and to focus on helping them through the terror of dying so suddenly (see www.therapeutic-touch.org).

During a treatment the practitioner assumes the existence of a human energy field (HEF) which is believed to be linked both to God and the cosmos and intervenes to enhance and balance it. The field can be depleted, blocked or unbalanced by injury or illness (G. Turner *et al.*, 'The effect of therapeutic touch on pain and anxiety in burn patients', *Journal of Advanced Nursing*, 28 (1): 1998). The HEF is worked on without the need for physical contact.

In this essay I want to show why this 'therapy' without a rational basis has captured the imagination of some eminent nurses, who are becoming quasi-religious practitioners of the twenty-first century, keen to promote its benefits to other nurses and, through them, to patients. The demand for TT in the UK is not consumer led but is promoted primarily by nurses. I will then argue that this is far from being a progressive development and that TT's promotion and integration into healthcare reinforces the notion that there is something wrong with scientific medicine. This does not benefit nurses, medicine or patients, but rather does each a disservice.

WHAT IS THERAPEUTIC TOUCH?

Delores Krieger, an American nurse and Buddhist, together with Dora Kunz, a clairvoyant and healer, introduced TT to postgraduate American nurses in 1975. TT is less well known to UK nurses than in the USA since cultural differences may have delayed its development and growth in the former country. Interest is developing in the UK, however. TT comprises phases that are learned sequentially but are dynamic and often performed concurrently and repetitively by practitioners. Self-examination is an integral part of performing TT. 'Beginning practitioners must learn to relinquish ego attachment. They must learn to lose themselves in the healing encounter'

(J. A. Straneva, 'Therapeutic touch coming of age', *Holistic Nursing Practice*, 14 (3): 2000).

CENTRING

This occurs before TT is administered. The practitioner's mind remains alert but becomes peaceful and calm through visual imagery or focusing on breathing, before going on to focusing on the recipient.

ASSESSMENT

This is the information-gathering phase of TT. It employs a tactile sensitivity of the hands for the purpose of determining the nature of the dynamic of the HEF. The practitioner perceives this as subtle sensations, which are highly subjective. In a state of health the patient as an energy field is perceived as a gentle, open flow from head to feet. In a state of illness the flow is perceived as congested and asymmetrical.

CLEARING

The practitioner moves the hands with the palms facing toward the recipient and at a distance of three to five centimetres over the clothed body of the patient. Gentle sweeping movements from head to foot are employed to activate the energy flow. Areas that are out of balance are sensed and mobilized. The cues picked up by the practitioner are extremely subtle and are typically described as, warmth, coolness, tightness, tingling, heaviness or emptiness.

BALANCING

The practitioner concentrates on drawing energy from the environment and directing it to the depleted areas of the recipient's field. The practitioner imagines energy entering his or her body, usually through the head. Many practitioners transmit energy to the subject through the visualization of colours. This conscious intent of energy flow is then directed to the patient's field through the practitioner's hands. After the depleted areas of the field have been energized, the practitioner's focus shifts to smoothing out the entire field, to help it feel symmetrical. Areas of congestion are adjusted by using the hands to shift energy to areas of deficit. The process is conducted over the entire body, comparing left and right in a head to toe direction.

EVALUATION

The practitioner uses his or her judgement to reassess the energy field to determine the amount of balance that has been achieved. The complete treatment takes five to seven minutes and can be repeated as necessary.

THE 'SCIENTIFIC' BASIS

Supporters of TT use scientific language to justify the practice. Former Dean of Nursing, Martha Rogers, developed 'the science of unitary human beings' as a basis for TT (M. E. Rogers, 'Nursing: science of unitary, irreducible, human beings: update', in E. Barrett (ed.) *Visions of Rogers's science-based nursing*, 1990). Drawing on quantum theory, she proposed that human beings not only possess energy fields, but *are* energy fields, which interact with the environmental fields that surround them. Human beings are considered denser embodiments of the energy that the universe is composed of. People schooled in the healing arts and other esoteric traditions are thought best placed to detect this energy. That evidence for the existence of a HEF has not been demonstrated is not a barrier to its acceptance as an explanation and basis for TT.

Although the origins of TT are steeped in religion, practitioners today do not need to believe in God. Nurses with an interest in the spiritual will find a welcome here, however, because of the current importance attached by some to spirituality in healthcare. TT is unacceptable to some religious people, who believe that only God should heal. A practice identical to TT but called 'auric' or 'pranic healing' is found in Western occult and Wiccan religions (D. O'Mathúna and W. Larimore *Alternative Medicine. The Christian Handbook*, 2001).

USES FOR TT

In response to a survey, British practitioners reported that TT could be used in most situations and for any number of conditions: on small ill babies, with fitting children, for acute and chronic pain, for people with HIV and ME, in first-aid situations and for psychological problems such as anxiety, depression, stress relief and hysteria (D. Lewis, *Nursing Standard*, 14 April 1999). These findings concur with results from clinical trials. Because TT is non-invasive, contra-indications for using it have not been reported. Similarities with magnetic healing have been noted.

In TT practitioners privilege the spiritual over the corporal and the organic and emphasize the distinction between healing and curing. 'Healing refers to a condition of harmony, a state of unity, ordered peace and connection' and 'to the emergence of the right relationship with or among body, mind and/or spirit: it is about becoming more whole' (L. Freeman and G. Lawlis, *Mosby's Complementary and Alternative Medicine*, 2001). Practitioners of TT are considered the 'midwives' of the healing process. Curing is used pejoratively by CAM supporters to describe the 'dis-ease' model of orthodox healthcare and refers to the process of eliminating signs and symptoms of disease.

TT also places a lot of emphasis on the intention of the healer. Some believe, as did Delores Krieger, that the pranic current (an ayurvedic concept of life forces and TT's active agent) can be controlled by the will of the healer. To be truly therapeutic TT is supposed to be deeply motivated in the best interest of the person who is touched. This seems very similar to the shamanic tradition 'which places great emphasis on the controlled and intentional nature of the experience, underlining that it is undertaken to gather knowledge and help healing' (M. Mooney, *Complementary Therapies in Nursing and Midwifery*, 2000).

PREVALENCE

Therapeutic touch is part of mainstream nursing practice in the USA. It is taught to nursing students in at least 80 universities. It has been suggested that as many as 50,000 nurses practise TT in the USA and Canada. It is also acceptable as in-service training for nurses, and the North American Nursing Diagnosis Association has classified 'energy field disturbance' as a legitimate nursing diagnosis for which nurses can prescribe TT. It defines TT as 'a disruption of the flow of energy surrounding a person's being, which results in disharmony of the body, mind and/or spirit' (T. Meehan, 'Therapeutic touch as a nursing intervention', *Journal of Advanced Nursing*, 28 (1): 1998).

Australia also has a thriving TT network. The first inter-continental conference of approximately 100 nurse healers was held in Adelaide in February 1999 entitled 'The Spirit of Healing – Myth or Reality'. A number of health professionals in the USA, in particular, view TT with concern and efforts to expose it as a metaphysical practice, without evidence to support its use, continue. UK critics are, in comparison, few.

TT is far from being a mainstream CAM in the UK and the demand for this therapy from patients is limited. US nurses promoted it to UK nurses at a London conference in 1987 as a new nursing technique with no harmful side-effects. Some British-based nurses continue to search for reasons to promote and use TT within the context of professional nursing practice and to justify its use in terms of benefit to patients. Supporters of TT advertize that the English National Board for Nursing Midwifery and Health Visiting (ENB) validated the first TT course, together with the former Manchester College of Nursing and Midwifery, in 1994 (D. Lewis, Nursing Standard, 14 April 1999). This is disputed by the ENB who report that validation was focused on armoatherapy and reflexology only (personal email correspondence). The focal point for TT training in the UK – the Sacred Space Foundation – continued to advertize on its website, until August 2001, that their TT courses were ENB validated (www.sacredspace.org.uk). The ENB does not keep a record of TT training courses and has not made a policy statement with regard to TT. It however recognizes the value of complementary therapies. A focal point for the teaching of TT in the UK is The Sacred Space Foundation whose director and chairman are both nurses. Fifty practitioners were registered with the British Association of TT (BATT) in 1999. The area of work of 23 practitioners who responded to a questionnaire then included clinical (mostly nursing), a GP and nurses in management or education (D. Lewis, *Nursing Standard*, 14 April 1999).

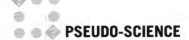 **PSEUDO-SCIENCE**

While scientific language is used to justify TT, actual scientific evidence to justify its efficacy is entirely absent. Practitioners are reluctant to engage in scientific tests to prove the existence of the HEF and rarely allow tests by people who are not TT supporters. Indeed, all Krieger's studies concerning the laying on of hands were conducted among supporters, at a theosophical retreat during

1971–73 (J. A. Straneva, 'Therapeutic touch coming of age', *Holistic Nursing Practice*, 14 (3): 2000). A nine-year-old American student, Emily Rosa, was allowed to undertake a study of TT for a school science project. She tested 21 practitioners to see if they could actually detect the energy field under controlled testing conditions. She asked the practitioners to guess whether she was holding her hand above their right or left hand. A screen hid Emily's hand from the healer's view to provide blinded conditions. Each healer was tested ten to 20 times. During the tests, the healers rested their hands, palms up, on a flat surface, approximately 25 to 30 cm (10 to 12 inches) apart. Emily hovered her hand, palm down, a few inches above the healers' hands. The healers' ability to guess the correct hand in 122 out of 280 trials (44 per cent of the time) was slightly worse than random chance. The report on the study concluded that TT claims 'are groundless and that further use of TT by health professionals is unjustified' (L. Rosa *et al.*, 'A close look at therapeutic touch', *Journal of the American Medical Association*, 279 (13): 1998). Scientific tests since then have been unable to demonstrate its efficacy.

In general, practitioners of TT concede that there are no scientific data to demonstrate the existence of a HEF, but because it is a working hypothesis, it is therefore valid. Straneva exposes the opportunistic and unscientific approach of TT supporters when she suggests:

> The underlying patterns detected in people's energy fields have been substantiated by healers working in tandem, but each healer's perception and description of subtle energy cues are highly individualised and based on his/her propensities. For example some practitioners see colours or images: others hear symbolic messages or inner voices during a TT encounters. Some healers feel kinesthetic sensations, vibration, warmth and/or pain, whereas others receive intuitive flashes that guide

subsequent action. The key to assessment of TT is avoiding rational analysis or judgement of the cues, and instead letting the practitioner's natural and intuitive inclinations take over.

('Therapeutic touch coming of age',
Holistic Nursing Practice, 14 (3): 2000)

The justification for TT rests on appeals to the value of 'intuition' and avoidance of 'rational analysis'. This is bad enough, but the fact that TT is dressed up in quasi-scientific language makes it all the more disreputable. Meehan, suggests that a working understanding of the framework requires:

> ... the ability to evaluate critically the on-going debate among quantum physicists about theories of non locality, and the debate among humanitarians and health professionals about the possible implications these theories may have for understanding the nature of consciousness and for promoting health and healing.

('Therapeutic touch as a nursing intervention',
Journal of Advanced Nursing, 28 (1): 1998)

She could, perhaps, have added that an ability to understand gobbledegook, liberally dispensed with accounts of the practice, is also required.

THE ACTUAL SCIENTIFIC BASIS

Many TT theoreticians use interpretations of quantum physics to endow TT with a 'scientific' veneer. According to scientists John Gillott and Manjit Kumar, quantum mechanics has been described as simultaneously the most powerful and the most intriguing physical theory of the twentieth century. Without it, most of twentieth-century science would not exist. Yet, they suggest, 'quantum mechanics also features prominently in an endless list of books which mix science and mysticism in the same blending machine' (*Science and the Retreat from Reason*, 1995).

References to physics in the TT literature are almost formulaic and serve to demonstrate a poor grasp of quantum mechanics by both its originator and followers. A profound but banal statement is usually asserted, followed closely by a nonsensical conclusion. Take the example of the lecture handout from Dr Snitcher (a doctor of medicine) of the Traditional Chinese Medicine Centre. We read that quantum mechanics (physics) is 'based on Einstein's proposition that all matter is energy'. It is hard to see how such a general statement as 'all matter is energy' could support any particular understanding of the body. The basic assumption made is that everything in the universe is made of the same sort of 'stuff'. Einstein's original contribution provided precise definitions of matter and energy and a mathematical relation between them. Proponents of the HEF never deign to discuss any of these 'details' although they actually constitute the substance of Einstein's work. This will hardly surprise anyone familiar with Einstein's work because, brilliant though it is, it is irrelevant to the subject under discussion.

TT proponents try to neutralize critics by suggesting that, however cranky their ideas and explanations appear, they are at least consistent with modern science. 'Science' is being used here not to provide a full explanation, but rather to try to suggest there is a space for TT in the unknown and half-understood (as with the idea that science is only now realizing the value of ancient wisdom). In this sense the discussion is implicitly about the limits of science. Although the form is to suggest that science can explain TT, the debate is in fact being used to suggest that scientific medicine is limited in its understanding. From this point of view, the more esoteric the physics, the better. The purpose of references to the least well understood aspects of quantum theory, such as the correct interpretation of non-locality, is to suggest that science still has much to learn and that it does not have all the answers.

But far from being consistent with physics, the idea of an HEF contradicts known laws. The HEF is not like any force field known to physics – gravitational, electric, magnetic or nuclear. If it were, it could be measured. The contradiction between known laws of physics and the proposed HEF is glaring. How does it interact with light so as to become visible to the eye? By what physical mechanism does it interact with the therapist's hands? To ask the questions is to reveal their absurdity. From the point of view of physics, post-Einsteinian or otherwise, TT is about as plausible as extra sensory perception or alien abductions.

Neither is it true that scientific medicine is unaware of quantum mechanics. The statement in the lecture handout that although 'Einstein's concepts have found acceptance in the minds of most physicists they have yet to be incorporated into the western biomedical model' would come as a surprise to biochemists who are now engaged in the 'molecular design' of new drugs. Over the last 50 years the understanding of quantum mechanics has made it possible to study in detail the way in which biological molecules interact with one another. This 'reductionist' approach is one that takes seriously the fact that we are made of 'vibrating atomic and subatomic particles'. Increasingly, the application of quantum mechanics where it is valid, on a molecular level, is in fact becoming more central to 'the western biomedical model'. Ironically, it seems this is the very approach that TT is most hostile to.

WHY IS THERAPEUTIC TOUCH ADVOCATED?

Nursing has undergone a crisis of confidence and of legitimacy in recent years. US journalist Sarah Glazer suggests that nurses have sought a professional identity that distinguishes them from doctors, yet provides equal status in a realm of their own (*Postmodern Nursing*, www.thepublicinterest.com, 2000). Some nurses have responded positively to this crisis by specializing, taking more responsibility, gaining more qualifications and even becoming consultants. A small but growing number have taken a different route and sought personal, professional and spiritual fulfilment in 'new' nursing and, specifically, in the adoption and practice of TT. According to the Chair of the British Association of TT, 'TT has brought a meaningful beauty into patient care' (N. Mellon, *Nursing Standard*, letters page, 7 July 1999).

The ascendancy of the therapeutic culture in society generally, with the elevation of emotion over reserve, is particularly evident within 'new' nursing. It believes that as a humanistic profession, therapeutic solutions and intervention as opposed to the curing obsession of medicine are in its and patients' best interest. This is evident from the number of nurses who train in CAM, ostensibly to offer patients a sensitive, holistic, natural, empathetic and spiritually based service. For some, TT represents a welcome rejection of a male monopoly of knowledge and of science and encompasses, instead, an appreciation of ancient wisdom. This has resulted in the favouring of non-western healing techniques over advanced medical technology and the pursuit of a less than demanding approach to science. They want to care and to heal, not to cure, based on the premise that these attributes are incompatible with orthodox medicine.

Steve Wright, a professor of nursing and holistic studies at St Martin's College, Lancaster, suggests that nursing has also lost direction and has entered a spiritual vacuum (*Nursing Times*, 23 April 1997). Some have developed 'energetic therapies', believing that illness is due to emotional and spiritual stagnation. They are encouraged to 'liberate' themselves, 'to come home to themselves', to spend time in the 'purposeful recuperation and nourishment of the soul' (J. Salvage, 'Journey to the centre', *Nursing Times*, 23 April 1997). Some get carried away completely by suggesting that if nurses worldwide were empowered with the healing potential of TT, they could help transform society as a whole (J. Sayre-Adams and S. G. Wright, *The Theory and Practice of Therapeutic Touch*, 1995).

Nurses Professor Carol Cox and Dr Anne Hayes have respond to criticisms made about TT by attempting to demonstrate that it generates positive clinical responses in patients in intensive-care units. They were, however, unable to show that there were any appreciable changes that could be ascribed to TT in heart rate, blood pressure, breathing rate and oxygen saturation levels in the small sample of 53 patients. They took comfort from patients reporting that TT helped them feel more relaxed and better able to sleep and concluded that TT may as a consequence benefit patients ('Physiologic and psychodynamic responses to receiving therapeutic touch in critical care', *Complementary Therapies in Nursing and Midwifery*, 5 (3): 1999). There is, of course, no way of proving that these psychological responses had anything to do with TT and could instead be ascribed to the placebo effect.

That the mind can have a powerful effect on the body under some circumstances is a well-recognized phenomenon in medicine. The placebo effect has a physiological mediator, usually opioids, but that does not mean opioids cause the placebo effect. A number of CAM supporters suggest, probably correctly, that much of their work with patients can be ascribed to placebo. Suggesting that placebo does not only have to be sugar pills – it can also take the form of hand waving, as in TT – Satel suggests:

It is very likely that TT recipients who feel better afterwards are experiencing the time-honoured placebo effect. This effect has rightly been called a window into the mind body connection, but it is by no means a magical phenomenon. In fact, any number of not so mysterious processes can explain why some patients experience relief after taking a dummy pill. Sometimes it's as simple as self-deception.'

(*PC, M.D. How Political Correctness Is Corrupting Medicine*, 2001)

Following a review of controlled trials for the proposed effects of TT (where she found little evidence), Meehan argued that because the placebo effect is so powerful, it 'offers nurses a natural opportunity to better understand and use this phenomenal function of human interaction to facilitate patient healing and well-being' ('Therapeutic touch as a nursing intervention', *Journal of Advanced Nursing* 28 (1): 1998). The implication is that nurses should not use placebo as a tool, since this elevates it to the status of a clinical intervention, which it is not. This could, of course, be profoundly dangerous to the well being of patients if offered instead of proper medical treatment: TT or cardiac resuscitation? TT or first-aid? TT or pain relief? The possibilities, and dangers, could be endless.

The charismatic personalities who promote CAM and TT are getting an unprecedented positive public response. The quasi-religious overtones of TT practice appeal to those searching for a spiritual meaning in life, but not wanting it from organized religion. The current obsession with lifestyle and with personal health maintenance is also fed by these practitioners. Patients also want what CAM in general promises them, which is not available or they do not want from orthodox healthcare professionals, doctors in particular, who they are encouraged to mistrust and view with suspicion: time, patience, trust, understanding, listening. Nurses, too, willing to capitulate to and capitalize on these developments, are fulfilling this need.

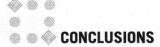

CONCLUSIONS

It would be easy to dismiss all of this as metaphysical nonsense because an HEF does not exist and that TT is a harmless preoccupation of some nurses. A number of criticisms can be directed at the practice however.

TT advocates like to promote the mystical notion that the universe is connected to people via an HEF. Manipulating this HEF is believed to help us to reconnect with nature and to live in harmony with it, instead of mastering and controlling it. Gillott and Kumar suggest that, in robbing humanity of the freedom to manipulate nature, by going with the flow as it were, they deny it choice and set limits on human ambition (*Science and the Retreat from Reason*, 1995). From this perspective TT incorporates a profoundly pessimistic view of humanity and about what it can achieve through science.

TT devalues healthcare that is based on objective evidence and science and pejoratively promotes the notion that modern medicine is mechanistic, reductionist and isolationist in its approach. It even blames medicine for causing modern healthcare problems. Promoting and practising TT reinforces the notion that there is something wrong with scientific medicine and undermines its coherence and strength. Dónal O'Mathúna rightly suggests that 'the world needs better application of scientific principles to all aspects of healthcare' (*Scientific Review of Alternative Medicine*, 1998). Precision, caution and scepticism about outcomes are vital components of scientific healthcare that have helped modern medicine become the success story that it is.

TT is a deception. Practitioners treat people with contempt by offering them less than the best healthcare available. Satel regales us with examples of TT practitioners who practise TT instead of seeking or providing proper medical treatment for their patients. She also suggests that TT is sometimes performed on patients who are asleep or comatosed, although without their consent. Parents, too, may be unaware that it is being practised on their children. This is abusive.

TT sells false hope by playing on the fears of sick, lonely and frightened people. The promise of relief can be powerful. Nevertheless, no matter how compassionate the practitioner's intent may be, according to sceptic and Chairman of the National Therapeutic Touch Study Group, Larry Sarner: 'The best caring and compassion by health professionals is for them to act knowledgeably and responsibly. Chasing will-o-wisps like TT, by wasting professional time and holding out false hope, can reasonably be considered cruel and inhumane' (*British Medical Journal*, letters page, 20 August 1999).

Nurses, too, are using patients as they cope with their personal or professional crisis, be it in a 'search for their spiritual self', 'embarking on a voyage of self-discovery' or 'coming home to themselves' (J. Salvage, 'Journey to the centre', *Nursing Times*, 23 April 1997). This is abusive, deceitful, self-obsessed and downright selfish. Nursing, according to Rogers, is a magnificent epic of service to mankind (M. E. Rogers, *An introduction to the theoretical basis of nursing*, 1970). Pursuing the logic of her 'science' within nursing does precisely the opposite.

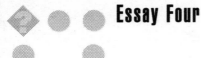

THE BEST OF BOTH WORLDS?
Michael Fox

Imagine. You walk into your bright, newly opened health centre. You are here to talk with your GP about your daughter's homeopathic treatment for her asthma. On your way in you meet your friend, who is just coming out with her toddler following a mother and baby aromatherapy session. After discussing progress with your GP you remember that you wanted to ask him about advice on the treatment of back pain for your spouse. He suggests that she refers herself to the open access, integrated backcare service (including chiropractic and osteopathy), which has just opened at the new healthy living centre.

On your way out you remember to return your book on *Why Integrated Health is the Future* to the centre's library and pick up another, *Better Eating*, which you had ordered the previous week. You pull your teenage daughter away from the interactive information station, where she had been looking for research on the internet about St John's Wort for her sixth form project on depression. As you leave, you see that the tai chi class for older people has started in the health centre's community room. This reminds you that you promised to get the timetable for your extremely stressed city neighbour on the centre's weekend yoga classes.

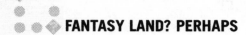

DEBATING MATTERS

FANTASY LAND? PERHAPS

All these examples do exist within the National Health Service, but they are scattered throughout the United Kingdom and are not available in one place. Tongue in cheek, the *New Scientist* recently said that 'perhaps complementary and alternative medicine is no more than a harmless fashion, like flared trousers' (May 2001) but the facts demonstrate otherwise. More and more people are using complementary and alternative medicine (CAM).

A survey conducted for the BBC in 1999 found that one in five British adults had used CAM in the previous 12 months. The most popular was herbal medicine, 34 per cent of respondents saying they had purchased it (although much of this was over-the-counter purchases from chemists and health food shops). The next most popular was aromatherapy (21 per cent) and homeopathy (17 per cent). Fourteen per cent had used acupuncture or acupressure, six per cent had used massage, six per cent reflexology and four per cent had used osteopathy with chiropractic attracting three per cent of the respondents. Another study, by Thomas *et al.*, estimated that 22 million visits were made in 1998 to practitioners of one of the six established therapies of acupuncture, chiropractic, homeopathy, hypnotherapy, medical herbalism and osteopathy ('Use and expenditure on complementary medicine in England – a population based survey', *Complementary Therapies in Medicine*, 2001). As a measure of comparison, the same survey highlighted the fact that there were 14 million visits to accident and emergency departments during the same period.

Within the private sector there is increasing interest in complementary and alternative medicine. A leading chemist chain has piloted the sale of complementary therapy consultations with its existing over-the-counter sales and is now developing plans to extend this initiative on a nationwide basis. One of the UK's major supermarkets has recently identified the sale of complementary medicines as a major potential growth area. In the leisure market, most health fitness facilities now offer a range of complementary therapies within their services.

A PASSING FAD?

Although there are limited data available, an extrapolation from the BBC survey just mentioned, suggests that the UK has an approximate annual expenditure of £1.6 billion consisting of both over-the-counter purchases and professional consultations. The study by Thomas *et al.*, suggests that £450 million worth of out-of-pocket expenditure was spent on the same six major therapies in 1998. This expenditure compares with an annual NHS budget of £50 billion. This level of spending on CAM is replicated in Europe, Australia and North America. For example, one study from the USA suggested a 47.3 per cent increase (over a five-year period) in visits to complementary practitioners from 427 million to 629 million with out-of-pocket expenditure on therapies estimated at $27 billion in 1997 (D. M. Eisenberg; R. B. Davis, S. L. Ettner *et al.*, 'Trends in alternative medicine use in the United States, 1990–1997: Results of the follow-up national survey', *Journal of the American Medical Association*, 280: 1569–75, 1998).

If the interest in CAM is being driven by fashion and the 'worried well' then an awful lot of money is being spent needlessly. Unless one entertains the unlikely notion that the 20 per cent of the population who are using complementary therapies are opting out of conventional healthcare, it is clear that what people are increasingly doing is integrating the different approaches to health. What people seem to want is the integrated provision, mentioned at the beginning of this essay. They want *the best of all worlds.*

Does it matter that people want both conventional medicine and CAM? Not, I would contend, to the patient who quite sensibly wants to use different approaches and methods to improve his or her health. But what about the different professionals? Here the 'pick and mix approach' does present challenges both to complementary and conventional healthcare practitioners, who may differ in their methods and, even more significantly, have different underlying philosophies about health, illness and the healing process. But, increasingly, as is clear from the evidence given to the recent exhaustive enquiry by the House of Lords Science and Technology Committee on CAM, there is more and more support coming from both quarters about the importance of being open minded about each other's abilities and perspectives. The select committee summed it up nicely when it said: 'We urge CAM practitioners and GPs ... to make patients feel comfortable about integrating their healthcare provision and to exchange information about treatment programmes' (House of Lords, *Select Committee on Science and Technology: Complementary and Alternative Medicine*, November 2000).

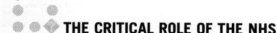

THE CRITICAL ROLE OF THE NHS

In July 2000 the Government announced its plan for the NHS: 'A plan for investment: A plan for reform.' It re-emphasized the NHS's core principle to provide a universal service for all, based on clinical need not an ability to pay. But access to integrated health is largely restricted to those that can pay privately for CAM and integrate it with more conventional services available through the NHS. The most recent study suggests that as much as 90 per cent of complementary medicine is purchased privately (Thomas *et al.*, 'Use and expenditure on complementary medicine in England – a population based survey', *Complementary Therapies in Medicine*, 2001). This may well mean that the more disadvantaged members of our community, who could most benefit from access to complementary services, are unable to do so because they do not have the funds and there is no local NHS provision. This is not an acceptable state of affairs.

Is this picture likely to change? Will there be local provision? If I had been asked this question even four years ago, I would have said that the possibility of CAM being made available through the NHS was low. But times are changing. Increasingly CAM is available within the NHS, a trend which is being driven by public demand. The response to the 1999 Foundation of Integrated Medicine and Guild of Health Writers award for good practice in integrated health suggested that provision within the NHS was far more widespread than expected. Homeopaths, osteopaths, reflexologists, acupuncturists, tai chi instructors, art therapists, chiropractors, herbalists and aromatherapists, it was found, are working alongside conventional practitioners particularly in primary care and also within hospitals. There are examples of integrated teams in mental health, maternity care and physiotherapy and specialist teams focusing on cancer, AIDS, multiple sclerosis and post-natal depression.

Integrated Healthcare: A Guide to Good Practice, a publication based on the integrated health awards, identified six advantages that an integrated approach offered to patients:

Clinical effectiveness of alternative treatments in many cases where conventional methods alone had not been successful; an extremely high satisfaction rate amongst patients; the availability of complementary therapies to many people who would not otherwise have the opportunity to use them, providing equity of access to care and increasing patient choice; the potential for significant cost-savings for the health service over the short and long term; bringing benefits to patients and staff, through the 'whole person' approach to care, and by creating a supportive, nurturing environment; improvement in staff morale and motivation, and a renewed sense of vitality to health services created through an integrated service.

(H. Russo, 2000)

What is the situation in the NHS more widely? In 1999, the Department of Health commissioned a survey across primary care groups responsible at the time for the provision of general practitioner and community health services for their locality, in order to find out which were the most popular CAM therapies being provided (J. Bonet, *Complementary Medicine in Primary Care: What are the Key Issues?*, NHS Executive, 2000). It was only a snapshot picture, but the more extensive BMA survey carried out at the same time reached similar conclusions about the prevalence of therapies within the NHS (British Medical Association, *Acupuncture: Efficacy, Safety and Practice*, 2000). The most popular was acupuncture followed by osteopathy, homeopathy, chiropractic and aromatherapy (see Figure 1). Interestingly herbal medicine, which is the most popular in terms of take up nationally (although this is largely product sales) is virtually non-existent in the NHS.

Closer to the ground, what do general practitioners who will be increasingly responsible for commissioning more and more health services, think about complementary medicine? In the same survey the DoH tried to find out. When asked whether they would commission complementary therapies, only a minority of primary care groups

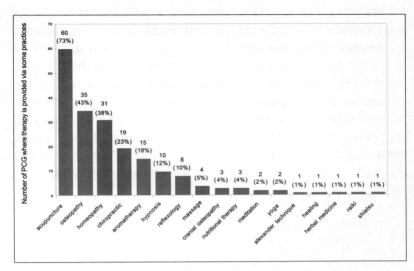

Figure 1 Therapies provided via primary care groups

(seven per cent) ruled this out as an option. Over 50 per cent thought it should be available within the NHS, while 44 per cent were not sure. Those primary care groups who answered that they would commission complementary therapies were also asked a follow-up question about funding. Nearly 80 per cent said that the NHS should either fully or partly fund it.

THE CHALLENGE TO COMPLEMENTARY HEATHCARE

It takes two to tango. If the challenge to primary care, which still provides the critical gatekeeping function to the National Health Service in the UK, is becoming more open about the possibility of providing CAM alongside conventional healthcare, then there are areas where the health service requires reassurance. If these concerns are not addressed, then integrated provision within the NHS and critically wider availability to those who cannot afford to purchase therapies privately will not happen.

In the same survey, primary care groups were asked about the key criteria, which in their view should underpin decisions about whether the NHS should commission complementary therapies (see Figure 2). These concerns ranged from the need to understand whether these therapies worked, whether they were cost effective and crucially whether they were safe and the practitioners providing them, competent.

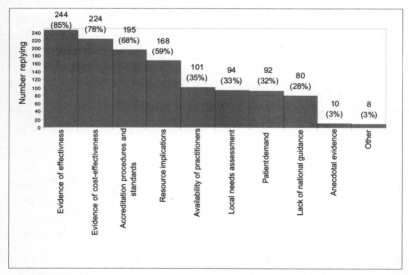

Figure 2 Factors important in decision making on complementary therapy provision

It is, of course, a chart that might confirm the public's prejudices about decision making in the NHS, with evidence and cost effectiveness out in front, followed by regulation and finance with patient demand towards the end.

It is not just general practitioners and health service commissioners who want to know whether treatments work; the patient wants to know too. There is a weak evidence base underpinning much of CAM. But of course the record of conventional medicine and its own evidence base is also at best imperfect. The advantage that conventional practitioners have is that they can at least more easily access NHS research funding than complementary practitioners who largely work outside the state system. Yet without evidence, the NHS commissioners and clinicians will not be easily persuaded of the necessity to provide complementary therapies.

This catch-22 was something that the select committee spent a lot of time mulling over, and one of its key recommendations was that there should be government action to provide some specific funding to pump-prime research and development. It was mindful of the example from the USA where the National Center for Complementary and Alternative Medicine has been established with protected funding (in 1999, US$90 million) to initiate a complementary and alternative medicine research programme.

It is essential that government does provide some support and the early signs are that, in its positive response to the recommendations of the select committee, it has recognized that it is essential to identify government funding for research into CAM (*Government Response to the House of Lords Select Committee on Science and Technology's Report on Complementary and Alternative Medicine*, March 2001). Quite rightly the public wants to know whether these therapies work, as do healthcare practitioners and managers. Although a search on complementary medicine on the internet will produce a vast array of data, it is difficult to work out what is authoritative and what is not. As a helpful first step NHS Direct, the Government-based health information service, has recently started to provide information on its website about complementary therapies, but considerably more work needs to be done so that patients can become better informed.

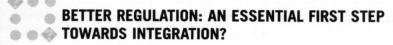

BETTER REGULATION: AN ESSENTIAL FIRST STEP TOWARDS INTEGRATION?

The common law right to practise medicine in the UK means that anyone can treat a sick person even if they have no training provided that the individual has given consent. In other countries in the European Union, for example France, this is not so and it is illegal for complementary therapies to be provided other than by doctors. The UK's liberal regulatory framework means there is a huge range of choice for prospective users of CAM; one of the Sunday broadsheets described 91 different therapies (*The Observer*, 8 July 2001). There are now, according to one estimate, over 50,000 complementary practitioners in the UK (S. Mills, *Professional Organisation of Complementary and Alternative Medicine in the United Kingdom*, The Centre of Complementary Health Studies, University of Exeter, 2000). The flipside for the public is that it is difficult to know who is competent and who is not as there is a bewildering array of qualifications. As the Prince of Wales said in 1999: 'Like conventional medicine, complementary medicine is only safe if practised by a skilled qualified practitioner and can be harmful in unskilled hands' (speech given to the Foundation of Integrated Medicine's conference, 14 May 1999).

Looking for a complementary practitioner is, therefore, not straightforward. The only sensible course of action is to rely on personal recommendations; the Office of National Statistics recently calculated that over 60 per cent of referrals to complementary practitioners was on this basis (Office of National Statistics 2001, unpublished data). But such an approach is not one that the NHS can easily adopt, not least because of the current well-publicized failures of regulation within the NHS highlighted in the Kennedy report on children's services at the Bristol Royal Infirmary and the tragic, unchecked activities of Dr Shipman in general practice.

For the select committee this was a key issue. Its recommendation, now accepted by government, made it very clear that only CAM therapies which were statutorily regulated or had well established arrangements of voluntary regulation should be made available on the NHS. Sound progress is now being made – chiropractic and osteopathy are now regulated on the same basis as doctors and nurses – and the other main complementary professions: herbalism, acupuncture, homeopathy, aromatherapy, body massage and reflexology, are taking positive steps towards the creation of single regulatory bodies.

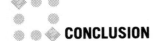

CONCLUSION

If the patient has anything to do with it, integration is here to stay. Both conventional and complementary practitioners are now clearly reaching out to one another and beginning to tango together. But as anyone who has ever tried it will know, the tango is a difficult dance to learn and partners need to be comfortable and confident in one another's abilities. It is clear, however, that the climate is changing; an editorial in the *British Medical Journal*, in its edition dedicated to integrated medicine, put it best when it said: 'Integrated medicine of today should be the medicine of the new millennium' (L. Rees *et al.*, 'Integrated medicine', *British Medical Journal*, 322: 119–20, 2001).

58

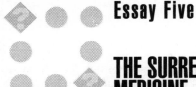

Essay Five

THE SURRENDER OF SCIENTIFIC MEDICINE

Michael Fitzpatrick

In January 2001 the UK Royal College of Physicians hosted a conference in London in collaboration with the US National Center for Complementary and Alternative Medicine on the theme of 'integrated medicine'. Two figures prominent in medical education in Britain and the USA explained that integrated medicine was 'not merely a synonym for complementary medicine': 'Integrated medicine has a larger meaning and mission, its focus being on healing rather than disease and treatment. It views patients as whole people with minds and spirits as well as bodies and includes these dimensions into diagnosis and treatment. It also involves patients and doctors working together to maintain health by paying attention to lifestyle factors such as diet, exercise, quality of rest and sleep and the nature of relationships' (Lesley Rees and Andrew Weil, 'Integrated medicine', *British Medical Journal*, 20 January 2001).

As a doctor trained in orthodox scientific medicine and practising within that tradition, I am alarmed at the widespread approval of the concepts of integrated medicine among doctors on both sides of the Atlantic. I do not believe that it is either possible or beneficial to reconcile mainstream medicine and alternative healing traditions. Furthermore, I believe that the shift of medical practice away from the treatment of disease towards a wider intervention in personal life in the cause of enhancing health and happiness is bad for patients, bad for doctors and bad for society.

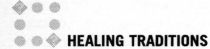

HEALING TRADITIONS

Alternative medical systems are so diverse that what they have in common is not immediately apparent (other than the fact that they are not orthodox medicine). However, if there is one unifying theme it is their commitment to a 'holistic' approach, which takes account of the patient's body, mind and spirit. Orthodox medicine is condemned for its mechanistic conception of the body, for its reductionist attempts to understand its function (and malfunction) in biochemical terms and for its interventionist style of therapy. By contrast, alternative approaches regard disease as a disturbance of the harmony between the individual, nature and the cosmos; treatment takes the form of assisting the purposeful attempts of the body to restore its natural balance.

If the fundamental principles of the alternative health movement sound familiar, this is because they are the same as those of the Hippocratic tradition which dominated orthodox medicine from antiquity until the beginnings of scientific medicine in the seventeenth century. Within this tradition there are broadly three sources of knowledge which provide the basis of clinical practice.

The first is revelation from some authoritative source, either divine or secular. For example, traditional Chinese acupuncture and ayurvedic medicine in India are derived from classic texts, mostly completed more than 2,000 years ago. More modern systems can be traced to charismatic figures, such as Anton Mesmer (hypnosis), Samuel Hahnemann (homeopathy), Daniel Palmer (chiropractic) or Andrew Still (osteopathy).

The second is speculation: this led early practitioners in a range of different cultures to theorize human health and disease either in terms of a small number of interacting elements, or humours, or in terms of the flows of energy or life forces through the body. Abstract theories or conjectures of this sort are common to contemporary alternative approaches. For osteopathy, 'subluxations', displacements of the bones of the spine, are the key to disease; in homoeopathy, the 'law of similars' dictates the selection of a remedy which produces a similar effect to any particular disease symptom.

The third source of knowledge is empiricism, the method of generalizing from the experience of observing numerous patients, classifying the clinical features of disease and studying the response to treatments. For example, healers using different plant preparations have built up a considerable body of knowledge about their effects (and side-effects).

Of these three sources of knowledge, in historical terms, the empiricist proved the most productive (for example, many plant remedies have been incorporated into modern drug therapy). However, doctors' capacity to observe and classify was constrained by the speculative theories that guided their selection of data. As the great nineteenth-century microbioloist Louis Pasteur observed: 'Without theory, practice is but a routine born of habit. Theory alone can bring forth and develop the spirit of invention' (R. Dubos, *Louis Pasteur: Free Lance of Science*, 1960). Scientific medicine emerged out of the empiricist tradition of observation and classification, but crucially advanced through the methods of induction and experimentation, developing theory by arguing from the particular to the general, elaborating hypotheses and testing them in practice.

Traditional healers turn ancient insights into laws of nature with eternal validity. For scientific medicine what was previously thought to be true has often been superseded by new discoveries. Whereas traditional healers express humility in the face of nature and deference towards established authority, practitioners of scientific medicine are sceptical and insubordinate, challenging divine authority and secular authority, questioning the evidence of the senses and the passive reflections of the human mind. 'Why think?' the surgeon John Hunter famously challenged Edward Jenner, the pioneer of vaccination, 'Why not try the experiment?' The historic innovation of scientific medicine was that it was open to critical evaluation and revision. Whereas alternative systems arrive in the world fully formed and complete, medical science is in a constant process of flux.

A common theme of recent official surveys of alternative medicine is the call for more research. The demand that alternative healing techniques be subjected to the full rigours of randomized controlled trials (RCTs), the 'gold standard' of contemporary 'evidence-based' medicine is often accompanied by the assertion that much orthodox medical practice lacks such scientific validation. Although RCTs are a valuable tool of research, particularly for comparing the efficacy of different treatments for the same condition, there are many areas of medicine in which they are unnecessary, inappropriate or unethical. They are highly unlikely to yield useful information about therapies such as herbal treatments when it is impossible to quantify the active ingredient and there is little understanding of the agent's mode of action. The application of sophisticated statistical techniques to compare the effects of homoeopathic preparations that have been so far diluted that they contain not a single molecule of the agent is simply absurd.

Medical science was scientific for many years before the advent of RCTs in the 1950s. In the years between the dawn of the scientific revolution in the seventeenth century and the emergence of effective therapeutics in the twentieth, it was the dynamic and open-ended character of medical science that commanded intellectual – and popular – support. In the early decades of the twentieth century the development of surgery and anaesthesia, antibiotics and immunization, and a host of other advances confirmed the ascendancy of scientific medicine over its ancient precursors and modern competitors alike.

The general trend of medicine up to the late twentieth century was to move away from superstition and empiricism and in the direction of rationality and definiteness. The unfortunate trend of the closing years of the century – expressed in the popularity of alternative medicine – was to return to pre-scientific conceptions and long-abandoned healing traditions. Given the backward-looking character of the vogue for alternative medicine it is remarkable that an openness towards such practices is today regarded in the medical world as signifying a progressive, even radical, approach. Why has there been so little questioning of what appears as a casual abandonment of the principles of scientific medicine that have contributed to the spectacular advances of the past century? To answer this question we need to consider the loss of nerve of modern medicine.

A CRISIS OF CONFIDENCE

In the last three decades of the twentieth century a number of factors contributed to a crisis of confidence in scientific medicine. These included problems within the world of medicine, a wider crisis of authority in society and popular disillusionment with scientific expertise in general.

By the 1970s, the hectic pace of medical progress that had been sustained through the post-war decades faltered. Infectious diseases had largely succumbed to antibiotics and immunizations (no doubt, clean water and better food played a more important role). Yet an ageing population now fell prey to the 'modern epidemics' of coronary heart disease and cancer and of chronic degenerative conditions, such as arthritis and diabetes, against which scientific medicine appeared relatively ineffective. New drugs (most notoriously thalidomide) seemed to have more side-effects than benefits and new surgical techniques (such as heart transplants) appeared to consign patients to a prolonged high-tech demise. Criticisms from within the medical world were gradually taken up by critics from without, creating a climate of opinion that was much more questioning of medical authority.

The breaching of the Berlin Wall in 1989 and the subsequent collapse of the Soviet bloc marked the end of the world order established after the World War II. Long fundamental divisions – between East and West, left and right – rapidly lost their force. The collapse of ancient polarities was linked to the decline of familiar collectivities (classes, unions, political parties, churches) and to the exhaustion of ideologies. The 1990s came to be dominated by preoccupations about the social and environmental dangers of globalized economic forces. In an era of lowered horizons and diminished expectations a climate of scepticism about all established forms of expertise became widespread.

'Doing better and feeling worse', Aaron Wildavsky's title for a symposium on the crisis of modern medicine in the late 1970s, struck a chord (*Daedalus*, 106, Winter 1977). It captured the paradox that, although by any objective criterion, such as life expectancy or infant mortality, people were living longer and healthier lives than at any time in history, an apparently increasing number of people were complaining to their doctors that they were feeling ill. At the very moment when medical science began to lose confidence in face of the modern epidemics, many people were now complaining of physical symptoms of fatigue, malaise and pain, for which it was often impossible to discover an organic cause.

Over the next two decades, more particularly in the course of the 1990s, the divergence between objective improvement and subjective deterioration continued apace. While the mortality rates continued to decline, anxieties about health became increasingly pervasive. Governments joined with medical authorities and the media to promote healthy lifestyles and to raise awareness of diseases, a process that took off in response to AIDS in the late 1980s and continued in relation to heart disease and different forms of cancer in the 1990s. Preoccupations with health intensified through an apparently endless series of the health scares (meningitis, cot death, MMR, sun/skin cancer, mad cow disease, mobile phones/power cables, thrombosis on the pill, thrombosis on long-haul flights).

In a period of increasing social and political insecurity, which encouraged an enhanced sense of individual vulnerability to environmental dangers, popular anxieties came to focus around issues of health. As the emergence of 'the worried well' as a familiar category of patients confirmed, the aim of promoting healthy living often had the effect of making people feel ill.

Feeling unwell, people turned to their doctors. This was partly because of the high prestige acquired by the medical profession through its association with the achievements of scientific medicine over the past century. It was also partly a result of the active promotion, initiated by prominent medical representatives and amplified through the media, of the GP's surgery as the first port of call in relation to a wide range of personal problems. The decline of alternative sources of solace and solidarity, such as churches, communities and families was another important factor. Unfortunately, patients who came with high expectations to consult their doctor were often disappointed. Presenting their intensely felt, but generally inscrutable symptoms, they found that many doctors were insensitive and unsympathetic. They often received inappropriate investigations and ineffective treatments, leaving them frustrated if not downright angry.

Disillusionment with orthodox doctors has encouraged the quest for alternatives. Insecure in their conviction in scientific medicine, doctors have adopted an increasingly conciliatory approach towards alternative practitioners. This is partly a pragmatic adjustment to the reality that many patients are seeing alternative practitioners, usually as well as, sometimes instead of, attending their GP's surgery. It also reflects a growing sympathy among mainstream doctors for various alternative approaches. Many doctors are now willing to refer their patients to alternative therapists; some welcome them under the same roof. Some doctors have sought training in acupuncture and homeopathy and medical schools now offer courses in complementary medicine.

The accommodation to alternative medicine is one indication of the loss of nerve of orthodox medicine. Another, perhaps more significant, indication is the transformation of mainstream medicine itself through the incorporation of the therapeutic ethos which has acquired widespread influence in society.

ILLNESS BECOMES A DISEASE

The tendency to interpret problems in society in emotional and psychological terms has grown steadily in influence over the post-war decades, most notably in the past decade (F. Furedi, *The Silent Ascendancy of the Therapeutic Culture in Britain*, forthcoming). This trend has emerged largely outside the world of medicine, but it has gained increasing influence within it. For example, it has become commonplace to discuss issues such as teenage pregnancy, drug abuse and crime in terms of the low self-esteem of many disaffected young people. The promotion of emotional literacy is widely recommended as the solution to educational underachievement, workplace conflict and even to communal and ethnic conflicts in Belfast, Bolton or Bradford. This therapeutic culture assumes a fragile and vulnerable individual self, whose stability requires the recognition and affirmation of others. The declining status of the public sphere (state institutions, political parties, social movements, voluntary organizations) has encouraged a retreat into the private self and intimate personal relationships. At the same time, however, high profile controversies over issues such as child abuse and domestic violence depict the private sphere as inescapably oppressive and dysfunctional, as a source of grave psychic damage. The emphasis on the psychopathology of personal life invites professional intervention, in the form of therapy and counselling. Not only have counsellors become a feature of virtually all modern institutions from schools and universities to workplaces and law courts, professionals such as vicars and rabbis, who have traditionally undertaken pastoral responsibilities, now seek training in the techniques of counselling. Just as every GP's surgery now has its counsellor, many GPs have acquired some competence in counselling. In this way, the therapeutic culture has, over a short period of time, become a major influence in society.

68

The issue of addiction illustrates the growing interpenetration of the therapeutic culture and the world of medicine (see M. Fitzpatrick, *The Tyranny of Health*, 2001). A sense of heightened individual vulnerability leads people to attribute responsibility for their behaviour to someone – or something – outside themselves. In this climate, the concept of addiction, the notion that a substance can produce a compulsion to act that is beyond the individual's self-control, has a powerful resonance. Alcoholism provides the model of a disease defined by uncontrollable behaviour which can be readily adapted to other activities deemed to be compulsive. Although it took the best part of a century for excessive drinking to make the transition from being regarded as a moral defect to being labelled 'alcohol dependence syndrome', the concept of chemical dependency was rapidly extended to heroin and, more recently, to nicotine. The medicalization of these behaviours has been facilitated by the development of medical treatments, such as alcohol detoxification, methadone and nicotine replacement, all of which are now available at a surgery near you. In the spirit of the therapeutic culture, official guidelines insist that all these treatments must be accompanied by submission to counselling. It is also striking that the world of treatment of 'substance abuse' provides a flourishing market for purveyors of various alternative therapies, notably acupuncture and hypnosis.

The redefinition of illness as disease has become the dominant medical response to the problem of unexplained physical symptoms. Thus people complaining of feeling tired all the time are told they have ME (myalgic myeloencephalitis), post-viral fatigue syndrome or, more recently, chronic fatigue syndrome. Those complaining of other symptoms for which no cause can be found are offered labels such as irritable bowel syndrome, repetitive strain injury, fibromyalgia, food allergy or even multiple chemical sensitivity. In familiar diseases such as tuberculosis or ulcerative colitis, even if the cause of the condition is unknown and treatment not available, a distinctive set of abnormalities of anatomy, physiology and biochemistry can be identified. By contrast, no characteristic pathology can confirm the new labels. Of course, the conviction that sustains support organizations for individuals afflicted with these labels is that medical science has yet to discover the nature of the underlying organic disturbance. For any observer who takes a historical or sociological perspective on the emergence of these novel illnesses, their origins in the existential distress of their sufferers is readily apparent (see E. Showalter, *Hystories: Hysterical Epidemics and Modern Culture*, 1997). The tragedy of the sufferers is their lack of insight into this process, a deficit that is reinforced by the provision of a pseudo-medical disease label.

The new diagnostic labels are descriptive rather than explanatory. Some – like ME – are obfuscatory, implying the presence of a pathological process that has not been confirmed in the vast majority of cases. Far from opening up the prospect of treatment, the new diagnostic labels merely confirm the hopelessness of the sufferer. In effect, the disease label validates and legitimizes the expression of incapacity in medical terms.

The proliferation of diagnostic categories in psychiatry reflects the tendency to apply disease labels to a wider range of social behaviour. Whereas in 1952 American psychiatrists recognized 60 categories of abnormal behaviour, by 1994 this had expanded to 384 (plus 28 'floating diagnoses') (American Psychiatric Association, 1994). Some psychiatrists have identified a much wider range of 'sub-syndromal behaviour' and people suffering from 'shadow syndromes', milder forms of conditions such as depression and anxiety, obsessional compulsive disorder and autism. The invention of new disorders – such as seasonal affective disorder, premenstrual dysphoric disorder and attention deficit hyperactivity disorder – reflects a further widening of the sphere of psychiatry and a blurring of the boundary between the normal and the abnormal. Whereas diagnoses in the past suggested the limited character of the condition, modern disease labels imply disorders that are unrestricted in the scope of the symptoms to which they give rise and in the duration of their effects. Post-traumatic stress disorder or recovered memory syndrome, for example, can be expressed in the widest variety of symptoms, which may arise long after the traumatic events believed to have triggered them.

The depersonalized character of traditional diagnoses allowed the sufferer to objectify the condition as something 'out there'. By contrast a diagnosis such as 'chronic fatigue syndrome' is inescapably personal in character. Every sufferer exhibits a different range of symptoms and there is no way of objectively confirming or monitoring the course of the illness. The net effect of the dramatic expansion in the range of psychiatric diagnosis is that, instead of conferring strength on the patient, bestowing any such label is likely to intensify and prolong incapacity. The proliferation of diagnoses and the tendency to apply them to increasing numbers of people reflects a profound demoralization of society and a deep crisis of subjectivity.

MEDICINE AS THERAPY

The effect of the therapeutic ethos on mainstream medicine has been to turn the problems of coping with the personal experience of illness into a major feature of medical practice. Contrary to the prejudice often expressed by advocates of alternative healing traditions, scientific medicine has made significant advances in a number of aspects of the psychological and subjective aspects of ill health. These include the emergence of the concept of 'psychosomatic' illness, from the study of work-related ill health and of casualties of warfare; the work of the 'hospice movement' in promoting the palliative care of patients with terminal illness; and the more precise understanding of the 'placebo response' resulting from the application of statistical techniques to the study of the efficacy of drugs. Yet in more recent years, the subjective focus of these once minor specialities has extended over wider and wider areas of medicine.

Thus, for example, the term 'psychosomatic' is now little heard as the concept of stress (arising from the workplace, traumatic experiences, adverse life events) has become universalized, leading to a wave of absenteeism and long-term disability. Palliative care has expanded into the provision of specialized pain clinics, dealing with diverse forms of unexplained pain (including headaches, facial pain, atypical chest pain, low back pain, total body pain). Although an understandable response to the growing numbers of sufferers from these conditions and to the difficulties of dealing with them within conventional specialities, the very existence of the clinics can be guaranteed to produce a growing demand for their services. While offering an ever-expanding range of diagnostic labels, these clinics mainly provide treatment with anti-depressants, cognitive therapy – and counselling. (Not surprisingly, they also increasingly offer a range of alternative therapies.) The placebo effect, in the past embraced by doctors who lacked effective therapies, but scorned by scientific medicine for confounding the study of its drugs, is once again welcomed (not least by alternative therapists) as a valid treatment in its own right.

The shift of medicine away from the treatment of disease to the alleviation of symptoms of illness in people in whom no disease process can be discovered has wider consequences. One is that, on the matter of doctors' skills in communicating information and empathy to patients, the pendulum has swung over the past decade from one extreme to the other. In the years up to the mid-twentieth century, when the scope of scientific medicine – at least in the provision of effective treatment – was limited, the capacity to display empathy and compassion for the sick was crucial to doctors' healing role. It is widely recognized that, particularly in the high-tech, hospital-based, surgical specialities that have been at the forefront of medical advance (such as organ transplantation, joint replacement, open-heart surgery) traditional bedside skills, even elementary civilities, have often become neglected. Among hospital physicians, who increasingly rely on sophisticated imaging and other investigative techniques and prescribe complex drug regimes, time-honoured 'physicianly' skills of history taking and physical examination have also declined in importance. Even among GPs, the capacity to prescribe powerful drugs, from antibiotics to anti-depressants, has tended to overshadow what appear to be old-fashioned pastoral skills of listening and reassurance.

Instead of the caricature of the surgeon who referred to patients according to the diseased organ he planned to remove and preferred to limit his contact with them to the time when they were under anaesthetic, we now have doctors who are systematically trained in bedside manners. The medical school curriculum has been reorganized to give the cultivation of what are deemed to be appropriate 'attitudes' equal status with development of 'knowledge and skills'. Formal training in communication skills has become an important part of medical training at all levels. Whether or not this training is effective in achieving its objectives (which may be open to doubt), its growing status raises concerns that training in the principles of scientific medicine and the cultivation of basic clinical skills is being downgraded. While the advent of social skills training is welcome to many who have experienced doctors who are ill mannered or uncommunicative, it cannot be regarded as a positive development in medical education and practice. It marks the loss of confidence of the medical profession in the advance of medical science against the continuing challenge of disease and an adaptation by doctors into the therapeutic culture that now permeates society.

Another consequence of the increased emphasis of medicine on the subjective is that it legitimizes the expansion of medicine into wider areas of the life of individuals and society. The advocates of integrative medicine welcome doctors' interference in 'lifestyle factors' and in 'the nature of relationships', although how doctors are qualified in either area is obscure. Yet GPs are being encouraged to intervene in issues of domestic violence, child protection, defective parenting and teenage pregnancy as well as in problems of alcohol and drug abuse. The result is that doctors are drawn further and further away from the medical sphere in which they have some expertise. Instead of practising medicine, they are taking on the roles of social workers, teachers and the police, assuming a more coercive role which can only prove detrimental to doctor–patient relationships.

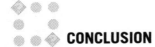 **CONCLUSION**

A recurring theme in the alternative critique of 'biomedicine' is that it remains in thrall to the rigid separation of mind and matter propounded by the French philosopher René Descartes in the seventeenth century. Cartesian dualism, the sharp distinction between a metaphysical human mind and a human body conceived of as a machine, is blamed for medical science's mechanistic approach to the body and its neglect of other dimensions of human individuality.

In response to this critique it is worth emphasizing that, for all its limitations, the conception of the human body as a machine has turned out to be extraordinarily productive. Apart from its encouragement to the study of anatomy and physiology, pathology and biochemistry, it also provided the imaginative framework for the emergence of transplant and artificial implant surgery nearly three centuries after this outlook was first propounded. By the mid-nineteenth century, Cartesian dualism was already being transcended within medical science itself, through Claude Bernard's conception of the organism as a 'living machine' with a 'milieu interieur' maintained in a dynamic equilibrium with the external environment. Through the work of Walter Cannon, Hans Selye, Macfarlane Burnet and others, the concept of 'homeostasis' contributed to the emergence of the specialities of endocrinology and immunology. The study of the mechanisms through which the human body regulates its internal processes and its interactions with the environment has contributed to a concept of a reflexive body that far surpasses the most sophisticated machine. These theoretical developments have been accompanied by dramatic therapeutic advances, from the treatment of thyroid disorders to the use of antibiotics against infectious diseases.

Yet, as the American neuroscientist Antonio Damasio has recognized, the ascendancy of Cartesian dualism has had some negative consequences (*Descartes Error: Emotion, Reason and the Human Brain*, 1994). By putting the mind beyond scientific enquiry and focusing almost exclusively on the body, it had the effect of delaying a biological approach to the mind. The failure of the discipline of psychology to become fully incorporated within scientific medicine reflects the slow progress in the scientific study of the mind, after the promising beginnings made by Freud and others in the early twentieth century. It is not surprising that speculation (psychoanalysis), empiricism (behavioural psychology) and mysticism (alternative psychotherapies) remain influential in this field. But, as Damasio argues, this is an 'area of weakness' in the western medical tradition that 'should be corrected scientifically, within scientific medicine itself.' His studies of the links between the perception of emotions and the processes of reasoning in the human brain indicate one way in which this approach can move forward. (At the same time he distinguishes between 'legitimate biomedical intervention' to relieve the suffering arising from neurological or mental illness, and attempts 'to deal with suffering that arises from personal and social conflicts outside the medical realm' which he regards as a 'different and entirely unresolved matter'.)

'It would be a tragic loss,' writes Prince Charles, perhaps the most influential champion of alternative medicine in Britain, 'if traditional human caring had to move to the domain of complementary medicine, leaving orthodox medicine with just the technical management of disease' (*British Medical Journal*, 29 January 2001). Here the Prince touches on what Abraham Flexner, promoting a medical curriculum based firmly on scientific medicine in the USA some 75 years ago, described as 'a curious misapprehension' that 'not uncommonly arises'. This was the view that the methods of scientific medicine were 'in conflict with the humanity which should characterize the physician in the presence of suffering.' But, as Flexner insisted, there was no contradiction between humanity and science – 'precisely the opposite':

For men are as apt to devote themselves to medical research and medical practice, because their hearts are torn, as because their curiosity has been piqued; and teachers, however intent on training students in the logic of practice, need not forget to inculcate, both by precept and example, the importance of tact and fine feeling. The art of noble behaviour is thus not inconsistent with the practice of the scientific method.

If the rise of alternative medicine reminds practitioners of scientific medicine of this basic tenet of their own tradition, then it has served some useful purpose. Otherwise, the only significance of its growing influence is that it reveals the stagnation of modern medicine and the loss of confidence in science that is pervasive in modern society, not least within the medical profession. What could better expose the demoralization of modern medicine than its reversion to theories that medical science transcended more than a century ago?

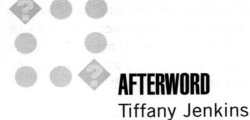

AFTERWORD
Tiffany Jenkins

The essays in this collection centre on different explanations for the popularity of complementary and alternative medicine (CAM) and the consequences of integrating CAM into medical practice. Contrasting opinions on these issues can be summarized as follows.

EXPLANATIONS FOR THE RISE IN CAM

CAM IS HOLISTIC

One argument for the rise in popularity of CAM is that it treats the whole person. Those who hold this view believe that the long, in-depth consultation patients experience with CAM is crucial to its popularity. Patients have more time to explain their situation and they are asked to explore wider issues in their lives. It is more personal than orthodox medicine. Patients are treated less like a machine, to be 'fixed', since consideration is given not only to the physical, but also to the emotional and spiritual dimensions of health. This argument suggests that the demand of the consumer accounts for the rise in CAM.

The relationship with the practitioner is equal under CAM because the patient plays an active role in the consultation through a shared identification of problems and solutions. This, it is argued, means that CAM is empowering to the patient. Orthodox medicine, by way of

DEBATING MATTERS

contrast, acts as if the doctors are the only experts creating a cold and unhelpful distance that consumers do not like. Many proponents of CAM point out that modern orthodox medicine is not as trusted as it once was. They feel that people believe orthodox medicine is unsafe and artificial. CAM by comparison is associated with a traditional and natural method and source that appears safer.

MEDICINE AS THERAPY

A different perspective is that there is a wider social explanation for the rise in popularity of CAM. With the collapse of old certainties, a widespread insecurity has developed in society, one manifestation of which is people becoming preoccupied with their health. The 'worried well' tend to attribute a general feeling of unease to a medical problem. CAM feeds off and encourages this preoccupation with health and acts in a similar fashion to therapy by soothing, but not curing. This explains the rise in demand for treatment that deals with emotional issues and offers little if no specific solution to physical disease.

Those who explain the rise of CAM in this way are often concerned about its effects. They argue that the solace sought in CAM only compounds these problems. It medicalizes social or personal problems. CAM may give patients false hopes that there is a treatment from a therapy or remedy that they can just swallow. In truth, if people are unhappy, they should instead try to solve those issues by addressing them head on. Understanding these problems as semi-medical or treatable with therapies will only mystify them and certainly will not solve them.

There are additional concerns about practitioners advising patients on matters of a non-medical nature. Consulting on personal lives or lifestyle could encourage doctors to intervene into areas of patients' lives they are not qualified to deal with. They would be acting as a social worker, priest, teacher or even like the police. This type of advice is not their area of expertise. It gives the doctors too much power of intervention into non-medical areas of patients' lives. From this standpoint, critical of CAM, medicine should concentrate on trying to treat problems that have medical solutions and not extend its remit elsewhere.

LOSS OF NERVE IN ORTHODOX MEDICINE

A different explanation for the rise in the popularity of CAM points to a 'loss of nerve' in orthodox medicine. It is argued that in the last three decades of the twentieth century a number of factors have contributed to a crisis of confidence in scientific medicine. These include problems within the world of medicine, a wider crisis of authority in society and popular disillusionment with scientific expertise. The very idea of a scientific method and cure has come under fire and is even doubted by some scientists.

Those that hold this view contend that those doctors and nurses who have embraced CAM and have grown sceptical of orthodox medicine are irresponsible to medicine and the patient. Orthodox medicine has a duty to uphold treatment that deals with disease and not waver nervously in the face of insecurity. This explanation propounds that the collapse of orthodox medicine is the significant factor in the promotion of CAM as a viable alternative or saviour to it. It claims that although there is demand from the consumer it is the failure of nerve in orthodox medicine that explains why there has been a dramatic change in the rise and acceptance of CAM.

THE CONSEQUENCES OF INTEGRATING ORTHODOX MEDICINE AND CAM

INTEGRATION OFFERS THE BEST OF BOTH WORLDS

Many who advocate integration suggest it would offer patients the best of both worlds. Patients would have more choice of treatment for their medical problems and would have access to more advice about improving their health. They could pick orthodox medicine for a medically treatable illness and mix it with CAM where desired. Most proponents of this view maintain that integration would improve CAM because it would ensure that it is professionally regulated. This would mean the patient could have confidence in the safety and the effectiveness of the therapies. A third reason put forward in support of integration is the beneficial impact it would have on orthodox medicine. It could help improve staff morale and motivation and give a renewed sense of vitality to the health service.

INTEGRATION MAY CONSTRAIN OR DILUTE CAM

Some who argue against integration are worried it could damage CAM. There are concerns that regulation would mean that if the therapies have no scientific base, they may be dismissed or encouraged to adapt, as they would have to fit into consistent criteria. It may be that fitting into the NHS will force CAM practitioners to cut down on consultation time. This would deny the patient the time for the personal and in-depth experience they should have. There is an apprehension that the recognition of CAM practitioners would elevate them to the position of an expert. It is argued that this could rupture the equal relationship between practitioner and patient that is so unique about CAM. This would re-create the distant relationship between doctor and patient in orthodox medicine which explains the turn towards CAM in the first place. A final concern about integration is that it would remove the 'alternative' in CAM. One of the attractions of CAM, it is argued, is that it is *not* mainstream medicine. If it looks like or is no different from orthodox medicine it may fail to continue to generate interest from consumers.

INTEGRATION MAY UNDERMINE OR DESTROY IMPORTANT PRINCIPLES OF ORTHODOX MEDICINE

Those who argue against integration from the opposite perspective contend it will destroy important principles of orthodox medicine. Integration brings a reversion to theories that medical science transcended more than a century ago. Opponents to integration from this point of view explain that orthodox medicine emerged out of the empiricist tradition of observation and classification. It crucially advanced through the methods of induction and experimentation, developing theory by arguing from the particular to the general, elaborating hypotheses and testing them in practice. For scientific medicine what was previously thought to be true has often been superseded by new discoveries. CAM, however, expresses humility in the face of nature and deference towards established authority. The CAM practitioners turn ancient insights into laws of nature with eternal validity. Incorporating these principles from CAM will destroy the gains of scientific medicine, which was once sceptical and insubordinate, challenging divine authority and secular authority, questioning the evidence of the senses and the passive reflections of the human mind. It is, therefore, a major step backward to integrate orthodox medicine and CAM.

This collection of essays indicates that there are strong opposing views on the explanations for the rise in CAM and contrasting opinions on the consequences of integration into orthodox medicine. While there has been little debate in the last 20 years about these issues, this collection aims to start a very important debate on the future of medicine. We hope that you have found this collection of essays an important step in opening up the discussion.

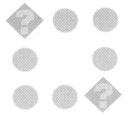

Other titles available in this series:

DEBATING MATTERS

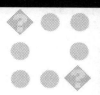

Institute of Ideas
Expanding the Boundaries of Public Debate

DESIGNER BABIES:

WHERE SHOULD WE DRAW THE LINE?

Science fiction has been preoccupied with technologies to control the characteristics of our children since the publication of Aldous Huxley's *Brave New World*. Current arguments about 'designer babies' almost always demand that lines should be drawn and regulations tightened. But where should regulation stop and patient choice in the use of reproductive technology begin?

The following contributors set out their arguments:

- Juliet Tizzard, advocate for advances in reproductive medicine
- Professor John Harris, ethicist
- Veronica English and Ann Sommerville of the British Medical Association
- Josephine Quintavalle, pro-life spokesperson
- Agnes Fletcher, disability rights campaigner.

TEENAGE SEX:

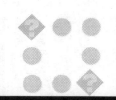

WHAT SHOULD SCHOOLS TEACH CHILDREN?

Under New Labour, sex education is a big priority. New policies in this area are guaranteed to generate a furious debate. 'Pro-family' groups contend that young people are not given a clear message about right and wrong. Others argue there is still too little sex education. And some worry that all too often sex education stigmatizes sex. So what should schools teach children about sex?

Contrasting approaches to this topical and contentious question are debated by:

- Simon Blake, Director of the Sex Education Forum
- Peter Hitchens, a columnist for the *Mail on Sunday*
- Janine Jolly, health promotion specialist
- David J. Landry, of the US based Alan Guttmacher Institute
- Peter Tatchell, human rights activist
- Stuart Waiton, journalist and researcher.

SCIENCE:

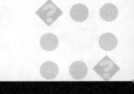

CAN WE TRUST THE EXPERTS?

Controversies surrounding a plethora of issues, from the MMR vaccine to mobile phones, from BSE to genetically-modified foods, have led many to ask how the public's faith in government advice can be restored. At the heart of the matter is the role of the expert and the question of whose opinion to trust.

In this book, prominent participants in the debate tell us their views:

- Bill Durodié, who researches risk and precaution at New College, Oxford University
- Dr Ian Gibson MP, Chairman of the Parliamentary Office of Science and Technology
- Dr Sue Mayer, Executive Director of Genewatch UK
- Dr Doug Parr, Chief Scientist for Greenpeace UK.

ART:

WHAT IS IT GOOD FOR?

Art seems to be more popular and fashionable today than ever before. At the same time, art is changing, and much contemporary work does not fit into the categories of the past. Is 'conceptual' work art at all? Should artists learn a traditional craft before their work is considered valuable? Can we learn to love art, or must we take it or leave it?

These questions and more are discussed by:

- David Lee, art critic and editor of *The Jackdaw*
- Ricardo P. Floodsky, editor of artrumour.com
- Andrew McIlroy, an international advisor on cultural policy
- Sacha Craddock, an art teacher and critic
- Pavel Buchler, Professor of Art and Design at Manchester Metropolitan University
- Aidan Campbell, art critic and author.

COMPENSATION CRAZY:

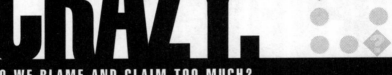

DO WE BLAME AND CLAIM TOO MUCH?

Big compensation pay-outs make the headlines. New style 'claims centres' advertise for accident victims promising 'where there's blame, there's a claim'. Many commentators fear Britain is experiencing a US-style compensation craze. But what's wrong with holding employers and businesses to account? Or are we now too ready to reach for our lawyers and to find someone to blame when things go wrong?

These questions and more are discussed by:

- Ian Walker, personal injury litigator
- Tracey Brown, risk analyst
- John Peysner, Professor of civil litigation
- Daniel Lloyd, lawyer.

NATURE'S REVENGE?

Politicians and the media rarely miss the opportunity that hurricanes or extensive flooding provide to warn us of the potential dangers of global warming. This is nature's 'wake-up call' we are told and we must adjust our lifestyles.

This book brings together scientific experts and social commentators to debate whether we really are seeing 'nature's revenge':

- Dr Mike Hulme, Executive Director of the Tyndall Centre for Climate Change Research
- Julian Morris, Director of International Policy Network
- Professor Peter Sammonds, who researches natural hazards at University College London
- Charles Secrett, Executive Director of Friends of the Earth.

THE INTERNET:

BRAVE NEW WORLD?

Over the last decade, the internet has become part of everyday life. Along with the benefits however, come fears of unbridled hate speech and pornography. More profoundly, perhaps, there is a worry that virtual relationships will replace the real thing, creating a sterile, soulless society. How much is the internet changing the world?

Contrasting answers come from:

- Peter Watts, lecturer in Applied Social Sciences at Canterbury Christ Church University College
- Chris Evans, lecturer in Multimedia Computing and the founder of Internet Freedom
- Ruth Dixon, Deputy Chief Executive of the Internet Watch Foundation
- Helene Guldberg and Sandy Starr, Managing Editor and Press Officer respectively at the online publication *spiked*.